THE MIGRAINE METHOD

The Steps to a Migraine-Free Life Through Science and Spirituality

ELIZABETH PRILLER

Foreword by Dr. Carri Anderson
Edited by Madeline Parise

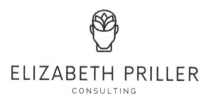

ELIZABETH PRILLER
CONSULTING

A published work of Elizabeth Priller Consulting

FIRST EDITION

Cover design by Elizabeth Priller, cover image by Getty Images Pro

ISBN 978-1-7369201-0-7 (paperback)

ISBN 978-1-7369201-1-4 (eBook)

UNITED STATES

Library of Congress Control Number: 2021909128

Dedication and Acknowledgements

This book is dedicated to God, for giving me the wisdom to translate my pain into purpose. *With God, all things are possible.*

I dedicate this book to my family. To my husband Jarrett in particular, for the ice packs, back rubs, and continual love during the years of my torturous migraine experience; to my daughters, Maria and Riley, for being patient with me when I was not fully present as their mom during migraines; to my grandson, Hudson, whom I love with all of my being; my brothers, Phillip and John, for always comforting me and willing me onward, but also encouraging me to take time to rest; to my sisters, for their unending love. With all my love, to my parents, Ellis David Chambers and Helen Maria, for giving me the foundation for my values of serving God, maintaining integrity, and always persevering in the midst of trials.

To the educators who nourished my thirst for knowledge and encouraged me to strive for excellence, most notably Mr. Ford, Mr. George Visel, Mr. Welp, and Mrs. Glenda Pecka.

And to you, the reader; thank you for trusting me and opening your mind to what I must share with you. I have poured my tears and my time into this book as part of my life's work, with the hope that it will help guide you on your path to freedom from suffering.

"And therefore, if the head and body are to be well, you must begin by curing the soul; that is the first thing. And the cure, my dear youth, has to be affected by the use of certain charms, and these charms are fair words; and by them moderation is implanted in the soul, and where moderation is, there health is speedily imparted, not only to the head, but to the whole body."

Socrates in a dialogue with Charmides, a young man with a headache.
(Plato, 380 B.C.E)

Table of Contents

SECTION ONE - THE INVISIBLE MIGRAINE: IT'S NOT ALL IN YOUR HEAD

SECTION TWO - METHODS TO RETRAIN THE BRAIN

SECTION THREE - A THRIVING LIFE

SECTION FOUR - ADDITIONAL RESOURCES

Foreword

"OUR CELLS ARE LISTENING TO OUR THOUGHTS." In what you are about to read, Elizabeth Priller answers all the questions that could be asked of this quote. A stunning journey not just through the brain, but into the mind and body of a migraine sufferer; Elizabeth connects them all in this exceptional work of education and self-exploration.

This engrossing work takes the reader on a journey of self-discovery that lights the way to healing from within, whether to heal migraines or other chronic pain. Travel through the anatomy of your brain and body, get to know yourself with Priller's easy-to-answer journaling questions, and finally find relief through multiple self-care methods. Employing better nutrition, breathing, yoga, and other techniques, Priller helps to educate and reassure with the help of ancient knowledge. She explains how, through positive self-talk and meeting your physical and emotional needs, you can begin your path to self-healing.

The Migraine Method is a necessary and enjoyable read for all physicians and healers, a great refresher and addition to the neuroanatomy and neurophysiology education from a root-cause perspective. From anatomy, to consciousness, to the exploration of self, this empathic work goes beyond explaining and healing migraines. Priller digs straight to the root of your migraines and helps weed them out for good.

Physicians and migraine sufferers alike will find this thoroughly researched book meaningful for healing, enjoyable to read, and an irreplaceable source for finding the true cause of migraines and how to naturally heal them with life-changing results. Elizabeth takes you with her as you find your path to healing through her method of finding the true cause of your migraines. Your body and soul will thank you for reading this healing treasure.

Dr. Carri Anderson

Preface

The root of all health is in the brain.
The trunk of it is in emotion.
The branches and leaves are the body.
The flower of health blooms when all parts work together.
- Kurdish Saying

I AM A LIFELONG MIGRANEUR who fully understands the frustration and pain of not being heard, of not finding relief, and of missing out on life. Over and over, I've faced the frustrating choice when debilitated with yet another migraine - "Do I push through, or do I stay in bed again, wasting precious time?" I know firsthand the pressure that the invisible disease of migraines puts on relationships, jobs, school, social life, and recreational life. I have suffered, and I want to use the pain I have endured to help you heal your own. Stay with me on this journey as I unfold the methods to living your best life free from suffering. My hope is that this book meets you where you are right now to help you continue your journey in a more fulfilling state of balance and wellness.

Health is a state of complete physical, mental, and social well-being, and not merely the absence of disease or infirmity.

- World Health Organization, 1948

The Migraine Method is not a cure. In our world today, people want to push a button or take a pill for instant relief of their suffering. Fair warning, this book is not a quick fix; instead, this book will help you peel back layers of imbalance to establish lasting changes in the circuitry of your body and mind. It is a step-by-step guide to a complete way of living that restores balance in your mind and body, reduces inflammation, and slows down cellular aging, all of which create a stable foundation to dramatically change your life experience.

From the age of 14, I experienced on average 20-25 migraine days per month, for over 20 years. Migraines were such a constant part of my everyday life that I tracked *migraine-free* days more than I tracked days with a migraine. After years of suffering and trying what seemed like every pill and potion, it was a traumatic event that finally influenced me to break away from my toxic way of living. From there, I started researching a way to free my life from the control of migraines. I developed and practiced these methods over a two-year period to address every area of my life that was causing imbalance in my health. And to my surprise, it worked.

Nowadays, migraines do try to "show up" if I slip off track in my daily practices. However, I have retrained my brain and body to not respond to the migraine as it once did, in the catastrophic, incapacitating, and violent way of days past. The migraine stops when I go back to the steps of the methods that my brain and body now recognize. On the rare occasion that I notice the twitch in my eye or the heat in the back of my head from not practicing the methods, I now know what to do to stop the migraine from going any further. I have not had to take any prescription medications or even an over-the-counter pain reliever for migraines in over two years which, for me, is a miracle.

I was skeptical about the power of healing. I had faced so many disappointments in new medications, devices, tests, oils, time off work - you name it, I had tried it. I had become a hopeless sufferer. What I have learned through this experience is that, as humans, we have faith in everyday things that we cannot see or understand; yet when it comes to the self, we do not have faith in our immense capacity to heal from within. For example, when we sit on a chair, we trust the engineer has properly constructed the chair to support our weight evenly. We start our cars and trust that they will take us to our destination, without fully understanding how they work at the most intricate level. We interact with and trust so many intentionally engineered processes in our day-to-day lives, and yet, we do not trust ourselves to be able to heal. This comes as no surprise when we consider just how much stress, anxiety, and poor lifestyle decisions are smothering us. We can't possibly heal - no matter our innate capacity to do so - if we are weighed down under insurmountable stress.

Heal Thy Self = Healthy Self

I fully believe that we possess the power of healing within ourselves. What holds us back is our tendency to bury that healing power beneath stress, pain, anxiety, toxicity, poor nutrition, and distorted beliefs. Our capacity to heal is only as strong as our relationship with ourself. How strong is your foundation? Where does your faith take root? What is written in the script you have been speaking to yourself? These are questions that you may discover answers to in this book, and through that discovery process I will encourage you build resilience for healing. The goal is that when stress comes, it does not cause you to fall or break into a cycle of suffering.

What you will gain

Throughout this book I will describe the theoretical causes of migraines, starting at the cellular level and moving into the electrical, vascular, and immune system pathways. When we understand what is happening in the brain, we can actively retrain the brain, a concept known as **neuroplasticity**. I will help you to connect your symptoms to the biological reactions that take place during a migraine. You will be able to identify which areas of your mind and body are out of balance, then take action to transform your physical and mental response to migraine triggers. You will learn methods to bring your body into alignment with the mind (the self) and the brain (the organ). Not only that, but you will recognize more precisely when and why your migraines occur, allowing you to smooth out inflammatory ruts. With consistency, you will be able to optimize your mental, physical, and emotional tenets of life, by removing the habits that contribute to suffering.

The Hopeless Sufferer

I recognize that starting anything new can be daunting, because fear often accompanies new experiences. Fear also squashes hope. In order to tap into your own biology and activate the healing within, you must have some level of hope. I know what it is like to feel hopeless; I spent over 20 years feeling defeated by migraines. Ultimately, I knew that I had to be desperate enough in suffering from migraines to examine every aspect of my life; that the only way I was going to remove the burden was to commit fully to addressing these areas and making necessary changes. This book results from years of research, trial, error, and success.

The methods in this book work most effectively with 100% commitment, but any effort toward rebalancing your life will move you toward wellness. The first question I must ask you is, "What is your realistic commitment level to improving your wellbeing?" Take time to ponder that question, because it needs to fit within the definition of your values and what is most important to you. Chances are, if you are reading this book, you may be at your breaking point with what has not been working, and you are ready for complete change - just like I was.

But I...

I will start right away by recognizing that not everyone has ease of lifestyle changes that are presented in this book. Perhaps you are the mother of a toddler who is struggling with a consistent bedtime; maybe you are a college student who is also juggling full time work. It might be that you are feeling so despondent and stuck in illness, the energy required to train your brain exhausts you just thinking about it. Perhaps there is considerable financial strain in your life. If any of these apply to you, consider me taking your hand right now and empathetically telling you that *I have been there*. I have been the person in all those scenarios I just described, and I value your time, energy, and resources.

I would also say this: consider the financial withdrawals you have already taken from your life in the form of prescription medications, doctor visits, missed time at work or school, or disability. Isn't it time to take your life back? Your lost time, lost money, and lost joy? Your life is sacred, and you deserve to be well. No price tag can translate your value. Honor yourself by taking this book seriously, as if your life depends on it- well, because it does. And, as you learn more about each of the methods to free your life and your brain from migraines, do what you can, one step at a time. As my mother often says, "When we know better, we do better."

How long before the migraines disappear?

I would love nothing more than to wave pixie dust over your head and remove your pain right here, right now. The reality is that change - real, positive change - takes time. Habits take time to unravel. Patterns take time to reforge. This book is not a quick fix. As I said in the beginning, it is a lifestyle map for those seeking enduring change.

On average, for every year you have been ill or suffering, give yourself one month for reestablishing balance. For example: I experienced excruciating migraines for 24 years. It took around 24 months of consistently following the practices in this book for me to feel my most well; to slow down cellular aging, reduce inflammation in my body, and stop the migraine cycle. Your results will also depend on other areas of your life, such as relationships, mindsets, nutrition, your overall health, your level of commitment to consistent practice, and any co-existing imbalances (in the form of diseases or disorders, such as diabetes, high blood pressure, autoimmune conditions, etc.). You are likely to see changes in your life within the first month, but don't stop there - the first uphill is only a small taste of how well you can feel by the end of your journey.

Over the next dozen chapters, you will learn about the science of the migraine brain, but don't worry - if you are completely unfamiliar with scientific concepts, my aim here is to accessibly present the principles. Concepts in the vein of biochemistry, neuroelectric wiring, gut bacteria, hormones, and DNA will be presented, to link the interconnectedness of the mind-body. Gaining knowledge about these concepts is going to help you understand yourself on an entirely new level. As the book moves into the methods of retraining the brain, you will:

- Learn how to finally sleep in a way that calms your mind

- Practice reframing your thoughts so that your cells begin to work for you, not against you
- Be acquainted with your DNA, discovering how genetics can be influenced to ward off the risk of disease

At the crux of the matter, where all these learning curves and processes converge, is **oxidative stress,** a prolific root of migraines, pain, and chronic disease. You will appreciate why this root is so important to remove from every aspect of your life. I will also introduce **Ayurveda** - the "other side" of medicine - revealing how to calm the migraine brain via daily practices such as a mindful breath in and breath out. This ancient practice is presented to help you identify and balance your Ayurvedic stress type for migraine prevention. Finally, the last section of *The Migraine Method* is the exploration of you; an opportunity for you to identify your core values, assess relationships that impact your migraine experience, and fine-tune your purpose as you move beyond the migraine and ultimately express your most authentic self. But first? We have some breaking up to do...

Open Letter to Break Up with Migraines

Dear Migraines,

Well, it's been a wild ride. I was young when we first met; I didn't realize the impact you were going to have on my life, the immense toll you would take. I have learned valuable lessons from you, it's true - but I am ready to move on. Breakups are never easy. There are reminders of you everywhere: in my bed, where I tried to sleep the thought of you away; in my bathroom, where I wiped away my tears from the pain you ruthlessly caused; in the top of my drawer, where medication upon failed medication used to lie, stagnant and utterly futile. You came into my life for reasons I don't fully understand, but I want to let you know loud and clear - from here on out, I am in control of how I respond to you and what I allow to enter my life. And, as my first step in taking back control, I ask you to leave. I will be patient as traces of you slip away, some harder to erase than others; but if you try to call or show up announced, I have plans to make sure you can't get in my head. Healing will take time, but I am committed - no, I am *determined* - that you will not be on the walls of my body anymore, that you will have not one single hand clinging to me anymore. We are finished.

Sincerely,

_____ (your signature here)

Introduction

"This book needs to be required reading for every medical student, healer,

and migraineur alike."

- Dr. M, Internal Medicine Physician

THE MIGRAINE METHOD IS A USER-FRIENDLY DEEP DIVE into the migraine experience through the magnified lens of the cells, the mind, and the end of the fork. This book is from my perspective: a migraine sufferer and Registered Nurse who, after 20 years of nursing practice and 24 years of suffering from migraines, studied to become a Certified Health Coach, Registered Yoga Teacher, and Ayurvedic Specialist to practice the "other side" of medicine. A four-month long migraine in 2017 left me desperate for relief. A painful but necessary ending in my corporate job gave me the space to refocus, re-evaluate, and reconnect my life, which resulted in a life free from the grip of migraines.

You will find among these pages my extensive mind-body research, as well as the trial and success methods that ultimately allowed me to live the migraine-free life I lead today. I will help you discover the mechanisms of how migraines express themselves in the physical and emotional body, as well give you the step-by-step whole-life guide that will help you tap into lifelong freedom from suffering.

In an intertwining of the complex processes of the inflammatory, biological, and electrical changes in the brain, you will discover how the mind-body-spirit connection orchestrates your individual experience with migraines.

The Migraine Method is a courtship of my personal experience, Western medical research, and traditional ancient holistic mind-body practices to help you retrain your brain and rewire the pathway to live a purpose-filled, high quality life. These methods will help you decrease suffering from migraines and guide you towards a sharper vision for living your best life.

The information in this book is not medical advice, but for educational purposes. I do not intend this information as a substitute for the advice provided by your physician or other healthcare professional. Results are specific to your own biology and commitment level and may or may not be typical. If you use the information for your own health, you are prescribing for yourself, and for which Elizabeth Priller and Elizabeth Priller Consulting assume no responsibility. I do not intend this information to replace or be a substitute for conventional medical care or encourage its abandonment.

I encourage you to practice what is best for your body.

SECTION ONE

THE INVISIBLE MIGRAINE: IT'S NOT ALL IN YOUR HEAD

Chapter One

The Person Behind the Migraine

You are what you believe in.
You become that which you believe you can become.
- Bhagavad Gita

AT ONE TIME OR ANOTHER, WE HAVE ALL BEEN TOLD to eat healthier, reduce stress, get sleep, and exercise to improve our health. The reality is that these changes are easier said than done; if it were that simple, no one would be seeking help for suffering. This book serves as not just the scientific *why* and *how* behind migraines, but also as a comprehensive blueprint for evaluating how each area of your life affects your migraine experience.

In every moment of the day, our brains use complex systems to monitor the internal and external environment, making small adjustments to keep us alive and well. Even when we think we are alone in our mind while lying in bed, driving to work, or sitting at our desk, our cells are paying close attention to the messages we give them. If you have been stuck in the negative mindset of "I will never get better," "Nothing ever goes my way," "I always feel sick," then your body will respond accordingly. If you are in a job that you dread, or a relationship that is weighing you down, your body will respond to the noxious threat accordingly. If you feed your body sub-par fuel, or deprive it of quality fuel, you cannot expect to be running on all eight cylinders.

The point of this message is not to be punitive or finger-pointing; in full transparency, I wish someone had opened my eyes many years ago to the self-sabotaging way I was living my life. I thought I was healthy because I ate salads and went to the gym. Unfortunately, the boundary line between wellness and illness is not always sharp. My mind was misaligned with my body to sustain wellness. I did not realize how closely married my cells were to my mind, or how receptive my hormones were to my words. The inner belief I had was "I am never enough," which is why I kept striving towards this invisible pillar of being "enough."

I worked a minimum of 12 to 16-hour days, said "yes" to more than I could handle, and allowed people, thoughts, and opinions into my life that were toxic to my well-being. In my childhood and teens years, I was navigating and processing trauma in the only distorted ways I knew how. In my early 20s, I under-ate, stayed in toxic relationships, smoked cigarettes, and drank alcohol. During my adolescence and again in my late 20s, I flipped my coping skills and became an overeater, eating foods that inflamed my body. For most of my life, sleep was last on my list, and only occurred if I made time, which was often in the three to five-hour range per night. Anxiety and depression were frequent visitors to my life, as well as anger, bitterness, resentment, and jealousy.

The boundary line between wellness and illness is not always sharp.

After years of suffering silently, a painful discriminatory incident at work shook me to the core, forcing me to reexamine what I was doing with my life. At the time, I was working on an administrative team as a nurse leader. My supervisor, who often acted imperiously, would berate me, publicly criticize me, and among other scenarios of high tension, the work environment became increasingly noxious. I stayed in this role for over two years, suffering from daily migraines, hives eruptions on my chest and arms, and recurrent anxiety attacks. My daily life bore a resemblance to working in a moldy, poisonous boxing ring with an opponent that could never be pleased and continually beat me into a corner of submission. I had become a shell of my true essence. I carried this burdened disguise home to my family. My relationships were unhealthy because I was exhausted, burned out, preoccupied with the past, and troubled about the future. I slept about four to five hours per night, and was stuck in a revolving door of physical, emotional, mental, and spiritual anguish.

The day I was forced to examine the way I was living was on a seemingly ordinary Tuesday morning at work. My supervisor was in a frenzy about a federal surveyor that arrived unannounced that morning. She turned to me and said, "Well, I met the surveyor. She is black, and she is mean, so maybe *you* can win her over."

I thought, *Win her over with what? Meanness, or blackness?*

I stood there completely stunned, as if someone had electrocuted my already fried nervous system with 10,000 joules of searing electricity. In that moment I did what I had learned to do to survive: I ignored the comment and continued working, pretending I was fine, all while I felt like I was shriveling bit by bit into a hole in the ground. For the weeks and months following this event, I developed welts of inflamed hives across my arms and chest each time I saw my supervisor.

I remember going home each day and asking myself, "Why am I allowing myself to be in a toxic environment that is slaughtering my wellbeing?" As people who are in survival mode naturally do, I was compromising my authenticity and my moral boundaries because I thought I had to. I endured the unrelenting stress of unrealistic work demands, the toxic conduct of others, burdens of relationships, and staying in environments of which I knew were not beneficial for me, but which I felt were obligatory. I wanted so desperately to maintain the status and stability I thought I was necessary at that stage in my life. I was fearful that I wasn't enough, that I had to keep proving my worth (to whom, I still cannot answer). I had tolerated situations that did not align with who I was. I realized I was moving away from my core values, a deviation which I believe produced disease in my life in the form of migraines and autoimmune diseases. I was drowning so deeply in illness I could barely see the light of the surface above me.

While we do need provisions in order to meet our needs, we must also possess the ability to reevaluate our situations and values to determine the impact they are having on our health. Chronic diseases do not develop overnight. A commonly referenced saying is that the bottom teaches us more than the top ever will; and I had to hit the murky and isolated bottom before I decided to surrender and come up for air. Once I hit my lowest low, I had no choice by to shift my lens to focus on eradicating the toxicity in my mind, body, and environment, and weigh in on how this toxicity plagued my experience with migraines.

Chronic diseases do not develop overnight.

Coming up for air and focusing on aligning my life was not an effortless task. I hit many stones of thought that echoed, "It's not working. I can't do this. What is the point of trying?" I wasn't sure what my goal was, but I knew that I had strayed far from my authentic self. I needed to clear out the cobwebs of what was making me ill and focus on calibrating my life for what would make me well again.

The seemingly precipitous departure of migraines was a byproduct of the gradual whole life changes I started to make, starting with the resigning from my corporate job. I was like you - I thought migraines were always going to be the immovable thorn in my side, affecting every part of my life for as long as I lived. In my mind, not making plans was easier than having a migraine ruin them for me. Where most women dreaded menopause, I looked forward to it; I had heard that migraines generally improved after reaching that stage of life.

Fortunately, my relief came much sooner - but not without its challenges. What I had to do was extremely difficult, more so than the time I escaped a headlock in Brazilian Jiu Jitsu practice against a man twice my size, or the 350-pound squat I had done a few years prior. I had to peel back deep layers to discover why my body was responding with incessant pain, inflammation, and other disabling symptoms of migraines. I have Type A tendencies, and I refuse to give up. I had to find out the *why*, rather than just battling against the *what*. *The Migraine Method* was born from this personal quest. I hope and pray that my painful experience, years of research, and subsequent freedom from migraines will help you to find a similar peace that I have discovered.

Pain

Life is pain management. From the first time we fall and scrape our knees, to our first heartbreak, life causes us to move from one painful experience to the next. Our lives should not be defined by pain, though pain is present and passing as we move through our journey. One way we learn about ourselves and our relationship with the environment around us is through affliction. A scripture in the Bible reads, "In every way we are troubled but not crushed, frustrated but not in despair, persecuted but not abandoned, struck down but not destroyed" (2 Corinthians 4:8-9). Pain is an experience that is entirely subjective; our reality is determined by the lens through which we perceive and interpret our life experiences. As migraineurs, however, we are often required to override this lens, taking the enervating and destructive experience of a migraine and equating it to a number between zero and ten. While this validates our pain to complete strangers, we know that it would take a much larger scale to encapsulate the pain we truly feel.

One of my most traumatic experiences with a migraine was one that mimicked a stroke, later diagnosed as a hemiplegic migraine. I woke up on a Sunday morning after my third day with the migraine and felt a tingling sensation on the right side of my face. Suddenly, I could not speak clearly; my right eye was watering, while my right arm felt limp and heavy. I was able to signal to a family member that something was not right, and I was transported to the local emergency room. Besides the physical symptoms I was experiencing, fear and anxiety rose in my chest. "Am I having a stroke? What if I ignored something more serious?" As the emergency room physician hurriedly greeted me, he asked me to rate my pain on a scale from zero to ten.

I murmured with slurred speech, "Twelve."

The doctor incandescently responded, "I said... *zero to ten*."

I bluntly replied, "And I said *twelve*..."

What I was feeling was so agonizing and complex that it felt far beyond a number on a scale. I couldn't convey the immense pain I felt in so few numbers. The doctor's stoic absence of a response was enough to convey that, despite my honesty, he didn't agree with my interpretation.

Clinical pain scales can be an effective way to quantify and measure a person's pain experience. However, if a 12/10 represents your pain experience, it is a 12/10. Just as a person who is 425 pounds cannot be accurately measured on a scale that only measures up to 350 pounds, sometimes our personal experiences with pain don't fit a fixed standard of measurement.

Author's Note: I started experiencing hemiplegic migraines after an ineffective anesthetic block in my neck for a shoulder surgery, also known as an interscalene block. When I experience tension and inflamed muscle spasms, it is almost always in the scalene muscles near where the block was administered. Although there has not been direct clinical evidence in my case to support the connection, the hemiplegic migraines started on the same side of my face and body as the interscalene block. A similar case was reported by Cook and Jones in 2008.

If a 12/10 represents your pain experience, it is a 12/10.

We relate to another's pain by comparing it to our own perception and experience of pain. For example, your toothache compared to my headache; if I have never had a toothache, I cannot possibly empathize with your nine out of ten toothache. The closest I can come to understanding your pain is by associating it with a different personal experience, such as comparable to a broken arm. The same rule applies to migraines - if I have never experienced a migraine myself, I can only attempt to understand your nine out of ten by comparing it to a different injury, like a broken arm. This cancels out a key difference between the two experiences: broken bones heal, but migraines return. The same goes for emotional or psychological pain. If you have lost your father to a traumatic death, I can more fully understand your pain since I, too, have lost my father to a traumatic death. We can empathize with someone if we have felt a similar pain.

If you do not change direction,
you may end up where you are heading.
- Lao Tzu

Interestingly, at no time during my 24-year migraine history did one person ask me about how my lifestyle habits (stress, nutrition, sleep, and mindset) might be contributing to migraines. I was experiencing stress due to my own choices, for instance, working multiple jobs, allowing negative people into my life, and exercising for two or more hours per day to distract myself from life. Most of my life ebbed and flowed from suffering to striving. For brief moments in time, I would experience a state of flow, feeling as though I was thriving in life. Then I would return home to be greeted by the cycle of suffering once more.

The Five States of Being

We are human beings, not human doings. As humans, we get stuck in a perpetual cycle of doing more, buying more, achieving more; dissatisfied and depressed, we wind up as contestants in the game of comparison. The inner monologue echoes "I will be happy when I...." convincing us that joy is conditional and does not exist in the present moment. Reflecting upon my own journey in this perpetual cycle, I have come to believe that there are five distinct stages of life which we all enter and exit over the course of our existence.

Amid a migraine attack, we enter the first state of being: **suffering**. According to the ancient text of yoga, the *Bhagavad Gita*, we suffer because we are faced with dilemmas and situations in life which threaten things that we love and hold the most importance to us. As migraineurs, we suffer because the pain and disability of migraines causes us to miss out on living healthy, vibrant, and engaging lives. When we release our attachments to the outer world, however - the perpetual cycle of needing and wanting more - we can begin to turn inward and free ourselves from suffering.

In between migraine attacks, as we anxiously await the next attack, we enter the second state: **surviving**. This is the space in which I spent most of my life, going from trauma to trauma and crisis to crisis, each gulp of air only just tiding me over until the next migraine hit. I worked over 60 hours per week for most of my adult life. There was no reason I worked that much, except for my self-imposed schedule which distracted me from dealing with myself. If I worked and filled up my schedule, I would not have to sit alone with myself. It was easier to keep a busy schedule to show the world how "busy" I was, as if being completely run off my feet earnt me an invisible badge I could proudly display. To boot, I allowed destructive people to infuse damaging mindsets into my daily self-talk. This is what happens in the state of survival: we are in auto-pilot mode, not giving much conscious thought to how our everyday choices and mindsets may affect our health.

The third state of being is **striving**, which represents the conscious act of identifying lifestyle habits that are detrimental to one's health or quality of life. This is the state where genuine change bubbles up to the surface, and the individual takes vital steps away from toxic behaviors or mindsets. Often, these steps are unguided; the figuratively drowning person grasps at floating life jackets as they pass by, hoping desperately with each one that it will be enough to keep them afloat. The striving person observes slight changes in the way they are living but can fall upon unstable footing if they do not have the support or guidance to help them transition into the next stage: flowing.

Former World War 2 prisoner Mihaly Csikszentmihalyi, one of the founding fathers of positive psychology, coined the flow state. In his research, he determined that **flow or flowing** is the state in which our ability to conquer a challenge is equal to the challenge, and we can enjoy the present moment (Seligman, 2018). To illustrate, think back to a time when you were doing something you loved, and time seemed to zip by in an instant. What were you doing? How did you feel in that moment? I recall one of the first times I experienced flow; the college nursing department head at the school I graduated from asked me to tutor nursing students. This was my first time speaking in front of a captive audience, and the three-hour lesson on the respiratory system seemed to go by in 20 minutes. I remember leaving that day saying to myself, "What just happened in there? That was amazing." This experience tapped into a part of my inner self that I didn't know existed, and eventually led me into my professional career as an educator. When actions are aligned with your inner self and you are executing your purpose, you are in a state of flow. A well-defined barometric indicator of your flow is the thing that lights you up with joy when someone asks you about it. In a flow state, there is no worry of failure, self-consciousness, or fear of inadequacy, and you have clear goals on your journey. Although flow is an incredible state to be in, I do not believe we stay in a state of flow. Flow is momentary and fleeting, but it sets the stage for us to thrive.

Thriving is the last state of being, best understood by differentiating between what it means to be buried, and what it means to be planted. In February of 2020, I started my vegetable garden from seed. I remember staring at the soil for weeks, thinking, "When are these seeds going to burst forth? Maybe I am just staring at dirt, and they aren't even growing." For a seed to sprout, the conditions of the soil must be at the right pH, temperature, with the ideal amount of sunlight, nutrients, and water. We are seeds; and packed tightly inside our innermost being holds our imprinted DNA and divine purpose. The state of thriving is a person who has a fair balance of health practices, regularly activates flow state, and is resilient to withstand the pressures of life.

Before we start exploring the science of the migraine brain, the first step of *The Migraine Method* is for you to identify these three key areas related to your state of being. Ask yourself these questions and write your responses in the space provided.

Suffering, Surviving, Striving, Flowing, Thriving

- What state of being have you spent most of your life in?

- What state of being are you in now?

- What state of being do you desire for yourself, and why?

Chapter Two

The Science of the Migraine Brain

Science without conscience is the soul's perdition.

- François Rabelais, *Pantagruel*, 1572

IF YOU ARE READING THIS BOOK, you likely understand from your perspective what a migraine is, and what it is not. A migraine is not "just a headache." Aching in the head is certainly a symptom of migraines, but that is where the comparison ends. The migraine experience is profoundly complex, varying in intensity, often accompanied by symptoms such as visual or auditory changes, nausea, vomiting, neck pain, eye pain, fatigue, numbness, mood or appetite changes, and others. The effects of chronic migraines extend far beyond the brain.

We recognize migraines as the second leading cause of disability in those under age 50 (Institute for Health Metrics and Evaluation, 2018). Migraine sufferers are three times more likely to be female between the ages of 18 and 44. The typical initial onset of migraine is near puberty, with a common improvement after menopause. Every episode of migraine can be a novel experience - even in the same person. For myself, I can differentiate between migraines that are caused by dehydration, versus lack of sleep or stress.

The history of headaches was first documented over 9,000 years ago. Aretaeus of Cappadocia, a 2nd century Greek physician, discovered migraines (derived from French and translated into Greek as **hemicrania**, meaning half the head). Interestingly, his foundational philosophy of medicine was that disease or disorder is expressed by imbalances in the body through **pneuma**, or vital air. (More to come on how the breath can alter a migraine in the chapter on *Yoga, Meditation, and Breath.*)

Unlike other conditions where pain is a primary symptom due to a single cause, migraine sufferers often report multifactorial triggers. The nervous systems of those without migraines generally do not hyper react to triggers such as odors, weather changes, lack of sleep, or dehydration. For example, my husband can miss meals and get less than 6 hours of sleep and not feel any different. Migraineurs know that this scenario would likely lead to a migraine. Recent studies also show that the highest risk of migraine development related to stress is around 18-24 hours after a stressful event. This proposes that the stressful event may not be what causes the migraine, but instead the aftermath of the stressful event such as lack of sleep, missed meals, fluctuating emotions, negative thought patterns, and general self-neglect that occurs after the acute stress resolves.

Types of Migraines

The most common migraine categories are **migraine with aura** (classical migraines that include symptoms of visual or sensory disturbances such as flashing lights), or **migraine without aura** (common migraines). Other categories of migraine include:

- **Abdominal**: presents with abdominal pain, nausea, vomiting; more common in children of families with migraine history.
- **Basilar-type**: a migraine that starts in the brainstem and produces symptoms such as double-vision, coordination and movement deficits, and dizziness.
- **Cervicogenic**: referred pain in the head from a source in the neck; caused by an illness or disorder, such as neck stiffness, vertebral misalignment, cervical osteoarthritis, or whiplash.
- **Cluster**: frequent attacks clustered together over time with periods of remission. Symptoms include runny nose, watery eyes, pain on one side of the head; thought to be more common in men.
- **Hemiplegic**: a rare migraine with aura that is accompanied by weakness or numbness on one side of the body (familial or non-familial types).
- **Ice pick**: sudden and severe headaches that may feel like a stabbing from an ice pick; no warning, generally only lasting a few minutes.
- **Menstrual**: migraines that occur at specific and predictable times of the menstrual cycle due to fluctuation of circulating hormones.
- **Retinal (ocular)**: may cause brief episodes of visual changes such as blind spots, flashing lights, or brief blindness that returns to normal.

- **Status Migrainosus (intractable migraine)**: a severe and unrelenting migraine that lasts greater than 72 hours, can be considered a medical emergency.
- **Vestibular (or migraine-associated vertigo)**: repeated dizziness that can also cause balance issues, with or without a headache.

Typical symptoms of a migraine include:

- Throbbing or pulsating on one side of the head that intensifies with position changes
- Localized pain in the eye, temple, forehead, or anywhere in the head or neck
- Increasing pain over 1-2 hours that, without intervention, would continue to worsen
- Symptoms lasting anywhere between 4-72 hours
- Other symptoms that may be present are nausea, vomiting, appetite changes such as food aversion or cravings, pseudo-odors (such as the odor of tobacco, cut wood, smoke, or cooking food), dizziness, tinnitus (ringing in the ears), allodynia (skin sensitivity or pain), numbness, tingling, fatigue, mood changes, sensitivity to light or sound. (Note: as the migraine progresses and once allodynia has occurred, interventions become less effective.)
- Observable assessments may also be present such as changes in heart rate, rhythm, or blood pressure, watering eyes, changes in pupil reactivity. One may experience *hemisensory or hemiparetic neurologic deficits* such as: inability to move a limb, facial drooping,

or numbness on one side of the face (such as in hemiplegic migraines).

Author's Note: Anyone experiencing a severe headache should have further diagnostic workup if the headache differs from their usual headache pattern or they develop new or abnormal symptoms.

Theoretical Causes of Migraines

As you've probably already been told, there is not a conclusive singular cause of the migraine. I remember my husband accompanying me to a visit to the neurologist; he bluntly asked the doctor, "Do you even know *the* cause of migraines?" to which the neurologist flatly said, "No." Researchers have identified suggestive cues to the migraine pathway: a combination of internal and external stimuli, resulting in an excitatory electrical storm, widened blood vessels in the head and neck (cerebral vasodilation), and neurovascular sterile (non-infectious) inflammation. An internal or external stimulus triggers a neurological domino effect, resulting in swelling of blood vessels that puts pressure on nearby nerves, which then sends electrical impulses to the most complex cranial nerve, the **trigeminal nerve** (cranial nerve 5, or CN5). When this nerve is irritated, it then activates the **trigeminal nerve system**, which can cause pain or sensory disturbance of the face, cheek, jaw, or eye. Activation of the trigeminal nerve system sends messages to the master control over the systems that maintain balance in the body, the **hypothalamus**.

How each person experiences a migraine differs, but the causes likely fall into one or more of these categories (see illustration on page 65).

Facts About the Brain

As I mentioned in my introduction, I want this to be an accessible resource; something you can read from a background of zero scientific knowledge and leave more equipped to tackle your migraines. If I were building a home, it would be wise for me to start with the blueprints before I jump in and start hammering away, right? So, rather than launching right into my methodology to living a migraine-free life, I want to start with the foundational science of the brain. Through it, you can better understand what's happening in that crucial space between your ears. Let's get into it.

The brain makes up three pounds of beefy tissue that occupies the space in our head. Imagine millions of connecting highways, billions of nerve cells, and thousands of neurons, all working to transfer a constant flurry of information. The folds (**gyri**) and grooves (**sulci**) are what create the peak-and-valley surface of the brain. If you've ever seen a pink cartoon brain, these structures are what inspire the squishy, spaghetti-like appearance. The brain spread out would cover an open two-paged newspaper. Nonetheless, there is much more to it than first meets the eye.

Gray matter takes up 40% of the brain tissue. This is what controls our ability to hear, smell, taste, feel, and see, as well as our speech, emotions, decision-making, and judgement. 60% of brain tissue is **white matter**, which is the fat-covered nerve highway that allows brain messages to travel at about 268 miles per hour from point A to point B. Every four minutes, a gallon of blood moves through the brain to nourish every cell, sending necessary glucose, oxygen, vital nutrients, and potent chemicals to and from the body.

The two sides of the brain - the right and left hemispheres - have distinctly separate functions. The **left hemisphere** is predominantly responsible for movement on the right side of the body and taking care of logical tasks such as mathematical equations, language, and critical thinking. The **right hemisphere** coordinates movement on the left side of the body. It is the primary brain area for expressing the arts, emotions, creativity, imagination, problem-solving, and memory. The brain is underdeveloped until around age 25; specifically, the **frontal lobe**, which is responsible for judgement, prediction, impulse control, personality, and social/sexual behavior. (This is why car insurance premiums go down after age 25 - you are less likely to recreate the car-jumping scene from your favorite movie when you can use forethought to calculate the potential consequences!)

The brain itself cannot feel pain.

Did you know that the brain itself cannot feel pain? You may be thinking, "Lady, I am sure I feel every cell of my brain on fire during a migraine attack!" I have been there - your brain certainly feels like the sole target during a migraine. The crazy reality is that the intense pain we feel is instead due to pain receptors in other areas, such as the nerves, blood vessels, and muscles of the head and neck; not the brain itself. **Nociceptors**, the pain receptors of the human body, are not in the brain tissue. Nociceptors are sensitive to changes in pressure, temperature, tissue damage, hydration, and chemicals.

Homeostasis - The Balance Game

Have you ever heard the phrase, "by the time you are thirsty, you are already dehydrated"? Our bodies are in a constant state of assessing information and responding with opposite reactions to maintain balance. This feedback loop monitoring system is a constant balancing act and critical for our survival. The brain is involved in continual cycles of information in, processing information, and sending action out. **Homeostasis** is the state of relative balance and stability between interdependent systems in the body - the yin and yang of the brain and body, you could say. For example, the body will work diligently to maintain an average body temperature of approximately 98.6 degrees Fahrenheit. As a person is exposed to prolonged cold temperatures, the body will begin to spontaneously shiver to increase body heat to maintain temperature homeostasis. On the contrary, the body will sweat in extreme heat to cool the body. We optimize our health when the body is performing in a balanced environment of internal, external, hormonal, metabolic, and chemical conditions.

Homeostatic reactions are essential to sustaining life and health. These reactions are automatic and predictable if the systems are functioning properly. In conditions such as diabetes, high blood pressure, autoimmune conditions, anxiety, depression, or migraine, the central homeostatic monitor may not interpret the stimuli accurately. Sometimes, the homeostatic monitor may overreact or under-react, leading to symptoms of disease or disorder. Allow me to illustrate: imagine you are driving down a dimly lit street and a moving object darts out in front of you. If your brain interprets this object to be a threat to your safety, you will probably automatically respond by swerving abruptly to avoid hitting the object. Within moments, having missed hitting the moving object, you will straighten the steering wheel, take a few breaths, release the brake, press the gas pedal, and continue your path. An *overactive* response would occur if you continued to swerve to the left after the perceived threat had passed. An *underactive* response would be no reaction to the object and staying on the same path, at the same speed. Such is an analogy for the nervous system: migraines can result from an overreaction of the stimulating areas of the brain, or an under-reaction of the relaxation areas of the brain. Often, one will experience symptoms of an imbalance in the form of disease or disorder when the body's automatic systems have exhausted measures to correct the imbalance.

As one would expect, the brain receives, interprets, and sends out signals to the body for survival. The brain is sensitive to fluctuations, such as lack of sleep, dehydration, temperature changes, and nutritive energy stores. In fact, the brain is the most energy demanding organ of the body, using about 20% of total body energy and nearly 25% of glucose in the body. The brain lacks the ability to store glucose, which is why it needs a constant supply of energy. Befittingly, this is one reason we cannot think clearly or experience changes in mood when we are overly hungry (commonly known as being "hangry").

Age and genetics will also influence homeostasis. For instance, an infant, a 17-year-old, and an 84-year-old will all respond to dehydration at different rates. This is because infants have small hydration reserves and a fast metabolic rate that leave them vulnerable to dehydration much easier than the 17-year-old, who has a robust and active thirst response center. The elderly person may be more at risk for dehydration because of a decreased thirst response, underlying health conditions, and a decreased fluid content in the body. External influences on homeostasis include food (energy), sleep, mental stress, brain chemicals, hydration, electrolytes, infection, hormones, blood sugar, and gut health, all of which send information to the brain about the state of balance in the body. Imagine - this surveillance is occurring nonstop during our life, while awake and asleep, from the moment we take our first breath at birth, to the moment we exhale the last of our breath at death. Take for instance how your body responds when you lack sleep. Sleep deprivation can enhance cravings for high-carbohydrate foods such as fast food, chocolate, chips, pizza, and other simple sugar foods. Cravings for these foods that stem from not enough sleep are in part because of the imbalance of circulating neurotransmitters such as serotonin and ghrelin, which are primarily manufactured in the gut. The brain senses a decrease in these important chemical messengers responsible for mood and appetite and sends the message to eat more to improve the levels of neurotransmitters. Our brain is constantly trying to keep the scales balanced.

External environmental triggers such as light, odors, weather, relationships, chemicals, drugs, alcohol, allergies, injuries, and pathogens will also influence homeostasis in the body; you can see this demonstrated through your body's response to a cut finger, for example. After the cut, the initial response is to jerk your hand away from the danger. The body then sends messages to the brain that an injury has occurred, and the brain in return sends messengers throughout the body signaling "all hands on-deck" for injury repair. Various responses from the circulatory and immune systems send their soldiers to clot the blood at the site, temporarily inflaming the area of injury to discourage bacterial growth and sending white blood cells to fight off any potential infection and encourage healing.

Another example is related to barometric pressure changes in the environment, which can trigger a migraine by changing the internal pressures of the spaces in the body, such as cavities, blood vessels, and nerves. When the brain perceives pressure changes in these spaces, inflammation and activation of the nervous system can occur, to "get away" from the offender. In this case, it may be the brain's way of satirically saying, "Get away from the impending storm and severe weather fluctuations and move to the Caribbean."

What you may notice about the various influences that affect homeostasis is that when they are imbalanced, some, if not all, have been proposed to induce a migraine. Think about your own experience with migraines. You may notice that lack of sleep, missing a meal, increased stress, or an impending thunderstorm may precipitate a migraine. Your brain interprets these changes in and around the body and attempts to elicit an appropriate response to correct the imbalance or remove the offense. Unfortunately, for those who suffer from migraines, one theory is that this system is faulty and overreacts to even the smallest changes in homeostasis.

Cortical Processing

The area of the brain that is most responsible for maintaining the complex framework of homeostasis is the **hypothalamus**. This miniscule region of the brain is approximately the size of a pea and positioned near the base of the brain. It serves as the master communicator between the brain and body and is responsible for the release of hormones. In a person who experiences migraines, changes in homeostasis consequently over activate the hypothalamus. This can lead to disrupted messages in processing of information. We refer to this mechanism as cortical processing.

Cortical processing is responsible for motor, sensory, and visual functions of the brain, primarily through the cerebral cortex. The cerebral cortex is the wrinkled surface of the brain that handles sensory processing (information in, information out), and is an area of the brain that is often affected by migraines. Prior to and during a migraine attack, there is a misinterpretation of stimuli, and this error can cause misfiring of pain modulating signals from the brain. The brainstem and cortex become hyperexcitable and overreact to the stimuli (such as over-correcting and swerving your car to miss hitting a leaf in the road). This repeated hyperexcitability of the brain and impaired processing is one theory behind migraines.

Current research indicates a distinct pattern from pre-migraine to the peak of the migraine, which reveals a blurred overlap of neurological, chemical, inflammatory, and genetic components that cooperate to induce a migraine. In the days or hours before a migraine attack, a person may experience mood changes, disrupted sleep, excessive fatigue or yawning, increased urination, neck or shoulder stiffness, or changes in bowel habits (such as constipation or diarrhea). Other migraineurs experience neurosensory symptoms collectively known as **aura**, which can include smelling faux odors, or **osmophobia** (an aversion to smells and odors), experiencing visual changes such as flashing lights, watering eyes, or **allodynia** (hypersensitive and painful sensation of the skin). I always knew when a severe migraine was on its way when I would spontaneously smell the scent of cooking bacon or raw tobacco out of thin air, yawned excessively, or if my right eye twitched.

After the peak of the migraine attack subsides, some people may notice a sudden shift in their mood, appetite, energy levels, or concentration. Studies show some individuals may even experience a sense of euphoria, whilst others may experience depression or the "migraine hangover." In my experience with migraines, I could confidently know the peak of the migraine was subsiding when I would start urinating in large amounts, my appetite returned ravenously, my vision appeared to be clearer, and the depressive mood lifted. For the next 24 hours, I would be in a semi-fog state, still struggling with speech, short-term memory, sluggish movement, and feeling "hungover," but the intensity of the migraine was on its way out.

The Brain on Migraine

Now that I have established how the brain prefers to operate to maintain the blissful balance of homeostasis, let's peer deeper into the brain during a migraine. Although experts in neuroscience have not narrowed down the exact cause of migraine, many agree there is a distinct domino effect in which the brain is in a state of hyperarousal in response to perceived threats. In the case of the migraine brain, these complex systems often overreact to triggers, resulting in three potential changes: dilation or widening of the brain's blood vessels, hyperexcitability of the nerves, and inflammation of the nerves and tissues of the brain. For this book, I will refer to these ripple effects as **VDI**, or Vasodilation, Depolarization (hyperexcitability), and Inflammation. Walk with me as we journey through a brain on migraine.

The brain is looking out for you
when you are not looking out for you.

The main switchboard of the brain, the hypothalamus, is the link between the nervous system and the endocrine system (which controls hormone release). As previously noted, the hypothalamus also controls body temperature, pain, oxygenation, heart rate, emotions, sleep cycles, thirst, hunger, sex drive, childbirth, blood pressure, digestive juices, expression of emotions, and balancing fluids and electrolytes such as sodium, potassium, calcium, magnesium, and water. This petite area of the brain receives various signals from throughout the body and then activates the pituitary gland to release certain hormones to help restore homeostasis.

Before a migraine occurs, the hypothalamus may receive messages of instability such as lack of food, extreme emotional stress, disordered sleep, or other chemical changes, and attempts to correct the imbalance. If we do not respond to the brain's subtle cues such as "drink more water, eat a meal, take a nap," the system is overstimulated and cannot recalibrate. For example, you may develop a headache and shakiness after not eating for several hours, which is the brain's way of saying "Hello, please stop what you are doing and give me some food so I can continue operating for your benefit." Or, you may have a sudden craving for a large glass of ice lemonade, which may be the brain's way of saying, "Since I can't trust you to stay consistently hydrated and give me the sodium, glucose, and water I need. Therefore, I am going to produce uncomfortable symptoms so that I get the fuel I need to keep you going." These may be harsh ways of simulating the brain's communication, but it gets the point across. The brain is looking out for you when *you* are not looking out for you.

As the brain responds to perceived threats or imbalances, stimulation of the trigeminal nerve occurs, which subsequently stimulates a release of inflammatory substances called **polypeptides**. These inflammatory substances such as histamine, Substance P, prostaglandins, tumor necrosis factor alpha (TNF-a), and calcitonin gene-related peptide (CGRP) flood the various areas of the nervous system, adding to the sensitivity of an already vulnerable brain. You may recognize the names of some of these substances, such as histamine or CGRP.

Author's Note: Occasionally, antihistamines are classes of medications that are used as off-label treatments to manage a migraine. This is one reason diphenhydramine (brand name, Benadryl) is used with other medications to treat an intractable migraine. The molecule CGRP, which is present in those with chronic migraines, has most recently become a target for newer injectable migraine medications. Later in this chapter you will learn more about what triggers the release of these substances, so we can attempt to remodel the pathways in our brain that trigger a migraine.

Cortical Spreading Depression (CSD)

The domino-effect theory of migraine stems from the release of inflammatory polypeptides (long chains of amino acids), activation of the trigeminal nerve, and a hyperexcitable cerebral cortex. The **cerebral cortex** is the covering of the brain and largest site of brain integration. The cerebral cortex interprets and processes information from short- to long-term memory, and is responsible for our attention, processing of information, language, our thoughts, and consciousness. We speculate that this is the area of the brain that is "us."

When the brain sends out warning signals and triggers a release of polypeptides (such as CGRP), the cerebral cortex becomes hyperexcitable, also known as **cortical spreading depression**. Cortical spreading depression is one theory of migraine development, since this is the electrical event that spreads electrical silence throughout the nervous system. To understand how this process works, imagine a runner getting ready to sprint the 50-yard dash. The runner prepares by kneeling and setting her toes on the line, waiting for the shot to start the push off. She is breathing deeply and preparing her body for the explosive start. However, she hyperventilates from overexcitement; she waits longer than usual, and her muscles tense and build energy potential for the take-off. Instead of the gun firing, someone in the crowd coughs, and she dashes ahead by mistake. 10 yards into the race, her muscles give out, and she collapses to the ground.

In this illustration, the runner builds up the energy to dash down the track. In the nerve cell, we call this **depolarization**, or the increased likelihood of cells to fire. In the brain of a migraineur, this process is exaggerated, leaving a nerve cell hyper stimulated to where even the smallest of triggers sets it off (such as the spectator's cough instead of the gunfire). Meanwhile, rapid changes occur in the fluid and electrolyte balance of the nerve cell, resulting in a large *influx* of water (H_2O), sodium (Na), and calcium (Ca^{++}). This positively charged group of ions *drives out* a large flow of potassium, hydrogen, glutamate, and adenotriphosphate (ATP). Researchers theorize that the sharp rise of potassium (K^+) could trigger an event of depolarization (a cell's readiness to fire) to nearby cells, resulting in further unnecessary firing of the nerve cells (like sparking other runners to prematurely take off at the finish line).

Cortical spreading depression (CSD) is the condition of the brain after the nerve cells fire prematurely and explosively, burn out quickly, and then have decreased electrical activity. This brain state is also potentially responsible for the aura symptoms experienced during in a migraine attack, that ultimately leads to activation of the trigeminal neurovascular system. Remarkably, the presence of CSD in the brain results in an increase in non-rapid eye movement (NREM) sleep duration versus rapid eye movement sleep (REM), which suggests the increased demand for sleep during and after a migraine (we will explore this more in the coming pages).

The Trigeminal Neurovascular System

As we continue to move through the migraine brain, you may start to recognize how changes such as barometric pressure, stress, lack of food, and inadequate sleep can trigger the brain systems to misinterpret signals and overreact in the form of a migraine. You may also recognize the pathway of your own migraine experiences as we reveal the intricate communication systems of the brain-body relationship. When the nervous system is working well, we rarely notice anything out of the ordinary. However, when this system under or overreacts, we notice symptoms of a disorder or disease - literally, lack of order and lack of ease. To continue, I will describe for you one of the most significant nerves in the brain and how it functions during a migraine.

A significant part of the neurological system involved with migraines is the **trigeminal nerve**, or cranial nerve V (CN5), which is notably the largest of the cranial nerves. The trigeminal nerve (TGN) exits the brainstem and branches into three areas of the head. The TGN provides sensation to the face, mucous membranes of the mouth, eyes, sinuses, and nose, and muscle control of the lower jaw. This nerve has two sensory branches (V1 and V2) responsible for sensation such as touch and pressure, and one motor branch (V3) responsible for chewing and movement of the lower jaw.

The first sensory branch of the trigeminal nerve is V1, which innervates the eye, tear ducts, skin of the scalp, forehead, upper eyelid, and has five branches of its own. When irritation of this branch of the TGN occurs, we may experience accompanying migraine symptoms such as crawling or tingling sensations on the scalp, pain on one side of the forehead, watery eyes, eyelid twitches, or drooping eyes. In my experiences with migraine, prior to the migraine starting I would notice tingling on the right side of my face, jaw tightness, and a twitch in my right eye.

V2, the second branch of the TGN, controls sensation of the upper teeth, gums, upper lip, mucous membrane of the palate (or roof of the mouth), and the skin of the face. Perhaps you have noticed tingling in your lip or face, tooth pain, or extreme salivation or dryness of the mouth before or during a migraine. If so, V2 irritation could be the reason.

The last of the trigeminal branches, V3, is a motor and sensory nerve that follows the jaw line. Have you experienced pain or tightness in your jaw during or before a migraine? This symptom may be a case of the chicken and the egg. When we are stressed, we tense and tighten our muscles, including the jaw. Check in with your body right now. Where are your shoulders? Are they pulled up towards your ears? If so, release them down away from the ears. Take a full, deep breath. Check in with your lips, jaw, and tongue. Is your tongue pressed to the roof of your mouth? Are your teeth clenched or is the jaw relaxed from its hinge? Are you breathing shallowly from the top of your chest or breathing deeply from your belly? The third branch of the trigeminal nerve may sense tension in the body which then causes irritation of the nerve, or the hypothalamus may notice the body or mind under stress and prompt the nerve to ignite. These mindful practices are part of the methods to calm the branches of the TGN, which communicate to the brain that all is well and there is no need for impulsive ignition of the nerve. Either way, it is important for us to check in with our body as not to further aggravate a delicate system that may be already hypersensitive.

Neuropeptides: The Chemicals of Inflammation and Migraines

When the hypothalamus perceives a threat or imbalance, the resulting chain reaction includes a flooding of neuroinflammatory molecules called **neuropeptides**. The hypothalamus activates the release of these chemical messengers to attempt to repair damage from imbalances. In the migraine brain, the release of these substances is premature or in unnecessary amounts. In chronic migraine, the repeated assault of these inflammatory molecules over time paves the faster than normal release, which can cause damage to the neurovascular system. Imagine repeatedly driving over a dirt driveway. When it rains, the ruts get deeper, and it is easier to get the tires stuck in the mud. Such is the migraineur's brain that has repetitive and often untimely release of inflammatory chemicals.

Neuropeptide Y

The first of these neuropeptides involved in migraines is **Neuropeptide Y** (NPY). This chemical assists in regulating our appetite, sleep cycles, stress resilience, sensitivity to stressors, thought processes, epileptic seizure activity, adaptive learning, and mood equilibrium. There are receptors for NPY in the trigeminal nerve ganglion (the central hub of the trigeminal nerve), which illustrates the connection between migraines and changes in appetite, mood, stress, and sleep. In fact, studies have shown that skipping meals may activate a release of NPY and change how the homeostatic system responds to energy stores. NPY is partially responsible for the noticeable increase of appetite during or after a migraine episode.

Calcitonin gene-related peptide

One of the most recent neuropeptides to gain notoriety is **calcitonin gene-related peptide, or CGRP**. This peptide is found throughout the body in smooth muscles, the brain, and the cardiovascular system, and is the most potent vasodilator neuropeptide, causing a widening of the blood vessels. Prolonged, chronic activation of the trigeminal nerve causes trigeminal cells to release CGRP, which mimics neurogenic inflammation of the brain.

Researchers have found that when CGRP is injected into someone with migraine disorder, it induces a migraine. Since CGRP receptors are throughout the body, the substance can affect multiple systems at once during a migraine. Most notable of these receptors are the **alpha receptors** of the peripheral (body) and central (brain and spinal cord) nervous systems, and the **beta receptors** of the enteric (gut) nervous system. When CGRP is released in the gut, it affects the motility, blood flow, inflammation, and secretions of the gut. New injectable medications that block CGRP have been at the forefront of migraine treatment, albeit with side effects such as severe constipation, increased blood pressure, and weight gain.

When high levels of CGRP reach the central nervous system, it induces sterile inflammation around the meninges (covering) of the brain. Areas of the brain that are also sensitive to CGRP include the hypothalamus, thalamus, insula, amygdala, and brainstem (more on the involvement of these brain regions with migraines in later sections). When an over sensitized brain hyper reacts to otherwise normal stimuli (such as lights, loud sounds, pressure changes, and other sensations) an inflammatory response is generated in the brain via CGRP. The sterile neurovascular inflammation caused by CGRP is what we interpret as the pain of a migraine.

Author's Note: In the chapter on oxidative stress and dietary supplements, I will share ways we can reduce CGRP levels naturally and reduce migraine frequency.

Pituitary Adenylate Cyclase-Activating Peptide & Vasoactive Intestinal Peptide

Next to CGRP, two critical neuropeptides are **Pituitary Adenylate Cyclase-Activating Peptide** (PACAP) and **Vasoactive Intestinal Peptide** (VIP). As the name suggests, PACAP is involved with the pituitary gland in the brain, which is the master hormone gland since it controls the activity of all other hormone secreting glands. When in excess, PACAP controls the secretion of hormones that suppress the immune system such as adrenaline, insulin, and cortisol. Normal levels of PACAP in the brain and spinal cord are neuroprotective and offer buffering of damage from decreased oxygen supply of the brain, such as in a stroke.

We consider VIP a potent anti-inflammatory neuropeptide which controls the balance of *pro*-inflammatory versus *anti*-inflammatory states of the body. Highest levels of VIP are found in the gut and the nervous system. A study highlighted by Arzani et al. in 2020 showed that in animals, VIP prevents the release of inflammatory molecules called cytokines (such as TNF-*a*) when there is inflammation of the nervous system. As discussed earlier, the release of cytokines such as TNF-*a* occurs when the brain senses an imbalance and activates the trigeminal nerve. This shows one more pathway (through the gut) to migraine development from a perceived imbalance or noxious stimuli in the nervous system.

VIP acts on the nervous system by widening blood vessels (thus lowering blood pressure), changing blood flow through the brain, and regulating the circadian rhythm (sleep-wake cycles). When we reflect on certain theories surrounding the cause of migraines, we know that some migraine brains experience a widening of the blood vessels (which is why caffeine can sometimes help ease a migraine by causing narrowing of the blood vessels). To no surprise, VIP levels tend to be highest in women with migraines. The highest measurable levels of VIP are early in the morning, which in turn activates and elevates **cortisol**, the stress hormone. I will highlight the relationship between cortisol, stress, and migraines in the chapter *Hormones and Biochemicals*.

It is important to recognize that activation of these neuropeptides occurs not only via the hypothalamus, but also through one of the autonomic nervous system tracks, the **parasympathetic nervous system** (PNS). The stimulation of these signaling molecules occurs in the presence of light, which impacts our sleep-wake cycles and quality of sleep. Keep the PNS in your back pocket for now as we will later explore how to bio-hack the parasympathetic nervous system to reduce anxiety, improve sleep, maximize digestion, and decrease inflammation to reduce migraine occurrence.

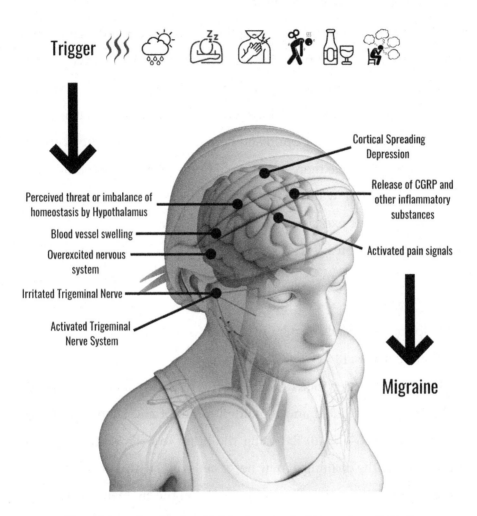

From trigger to migraine. Original anatomical image from Getty Images.

Brain-Derived Neurotrophic Factor

Another vitally protective neuropeptide is **brain-derived neurotrophic factor**, or BDNF. BDNF provides a nourishing and restorative wash for the brain to help with healing of damaged tissue. After an episode of cortical spreading depression during a migraine, BDNF acts comparable to a massage, to soothe the brain and help form new connections after the electrical storm. While there is not a pill or supplement that can increase BDNF, one natural way to increase BDNF levels is through exercise, specifically aerobic exercise. Aerobic exercise that elevates the heart rate for at least 10 minutes (such as running, biking, dancing, hiking, skiing, kickboxing, or team sports), followed by a skill-based exercise (such as studying or learning a new skill), has been shown to increase BDNF levels and help the brain cells form new connections. As exercise intensity and duration increases, BDNF levels also increase.

In a phenomenon called **neuroplasticity**, scientists have found that the brain can be molded and remolded to adapt and change depending on what we expose it to. Exposing the brain to exercise helps support **neurogenesis** (the forming of new nerve cells) in the **hippocampus**, which is the center for spatial processing and long-term memory retention. BDNF supports a healthy brain and may even help ward off memory loss. This protective substance is also the reason for our improved well-being and mood after we exercise. Aerobic exercise also increases the size and maximizes the function of the hippocampus. What a golden opportunity it is to learn a new language or skill after you get back from the gym!

Other Critical Areas of the Migraine Brain

The **insula**, Latin for "island," is a lesser-known cornerstone of the cerebral cortex that processes basic survival sensory input such as taste, sensation, pain, pressure, sounds, light, and movement. The insula also regulates the **sympathetic nervous system** (automatic processes related to fight or flight) and the **parasympathetic nervous system** (automatic processes related to rest and digest) and plays a noteworthy role in regulation of the immune system.

We postulate the insula to be our observation of "self." If you paused right now and were to describe how you feel, who you are, what you are thinking about, and how your experiences have molded you, you would find these sensations tucked away in the insula. The experience of knowing and sensing what is going on inside your body and how you feel we refer to as **interoception**. The insula encapsulates our innermost feelings, which then translate into thoughts, reasoning, beliefs, actions, and behaviors. It can be challenging to express to the outside world what is only visible and perceived by us. To illustrate how the insula works to connect our emotions to our physical health, take, for instance, this fictional character, "Robin".

Case Study Example

Robin is a 35-year-old woman who lives with her boyfriend of three years. She grew up in rural Iowa, but for the last five years has lived in a condo in the bustling city of Indianapolis. She moved to the city after landing her first job as a senior accountant at a distinguished financial firm. Robin feels she is successful in her work, but a train wreck at home. She spends hours a day figuratively "holding her breath" to maintain a persona of having it all together. When she gets home, she collapses in front of the TV with a nightly bottle of wine, an escape from her stressful job.

Robin wants to have children, but she knows that her boyfriend is not father-figure material. She finds that she tends to stick out unfulfilling relationships, jobs, and even hairstyles just to keep the peace, when on the inside she is stressed, unhappy, and overweight. She habitually feels stuck. Robin has also been suffering from migraines since she was 15, along with a new diagnosis of diabetes and high blood pressure.

Her daily self-talk echoes, "I don't know why I even bothered with grad school. I'm not even happy at this dog-eat-dog firm. I'll never pay off all this debt. I am so sick and tired of doing things I don't want to. Ugh, and these thighs. Who in the world would ever take me seriously with this extra 40 pounds I am carrying around? I can't even control what I eat, let alone try to exercise. Sleep? What sleep? Every night I just lay there and toss and turn until about 2 am. Then my mother wants to lecture me that if I just exercised it would be better. It is too late now. I am halfway to 70. And I am already overweight and diabetic now, too. Damn it, here comes another migraine. My body is so stupid! Where is my ibuprofen…"

This is a raw example of a woman dealing with chronic stress, being overweight, and feeling unhappy and unfulfilled in her life. She is experiencing disturbances in her body and stuffing of emotions, manifesting in the form of migraines, diabetes, and high blood pressure. This story shows just one of many ways that a thought or feeling can turn into a belief, which then turns into a choice, then a pattern, and finally, into a learned behavior. The snowball effect of stress, thoughts, emotions, choices, and behaviors directly influence our health. As put so laconically by Deepak Chopra, "Our cells are listening to our thoughts." Here, the insula is monitoring this woman's feelings and thoughts, and sending information to the body about the situations in her world. In a system that may already be exhausted and imbalanced, these automatic responses are less than desirable for wellbeing. The insula, in cooperation with other neurological areas, is monitoring what we see, hear, feel, taste, smell, and turning these experiences into biological responses.

System Shut Down

Think about when you experience the onset of a migraine. Perhaps it is the nausea, light sensitivity, or pain over the eye that signals to you the onset of a migraine. I recall nearly every time a migraine would start, I would say to myself or to whoever would listen, "I cannot believe this is happening. Another migraine. I have so much to do! I can't sit here and sleep and waste my life! I am so tired of losing my life over a stupid headache that I have no control over." I remember instantly feeling sad, regretful, and depressed, and almost always the migraine would continue its course no matter what medications I took.

In one season of my life in 2017, I had several major life changes that happened in rapid succession which overloaded my already fragile system. I moved to a new town where I knew no one except my new fiancé, uprooted my kids from their school, left a community I had developed deep roots in, was working two jobs 14-16 hour per day, trying to sell my home, and was a full-time graduate student for my master's in nursing education. In Spring of 2017, I had an inexorable four-month long migraine with less than 4-5 days of relief during those months. I was suffering beyond explanation. Still, somehow, I just kept telling myself, *If I keep going, I will get through it, and it will pass.* I will never forget the day my nervous system completely shut down: May 9, 2017.

I was heading into the school where I was teaching, finally having eased my work schedule back to a manageable eight-to-ten-hour workday. I was feeling an unacquainted sense of calm that morning. I was proud of myself, as I had finally taken back some control and balance in my schedule. As I was walking towards the school, carrying my 1,800-page pathophysiology book in hand to study over my lunch break, I reached my hand towards the building door. The moment my hand met the door handle, it was as if I had been electrocuted. Immediately my head spun, my vision became blurry, and I overheated profusely. I became so feverish, I stumbled to find a faucet to splash myself with water. The disequilibrium continued, and I could barely stand up straight. My ears rang; the wave of repugnance hit me. I vomited right in the hallway of the school. As I struggled to reach my office, every attempt at speech was slurred. I just needed to alert someone that I was in trouble.

I was able to stagger onto the lab hospital bed. Luck would have it that one of my students came early to class; she had plans to go to school to become an emergency medicine physician, so my sudden event quickly became suitable practice for her. I was able to direct her on what to do (help me lie down with my feet up, place ice packs around my neck and arms, check my blood pressure, and call my husband). You may be thinking - "Why didn't you call 9-1-1?"

Well, even in that blurry, spinning room, I knew what was happening. Added to my stubbornness of not wanting to visit an emergency room, I wanted to wait to see if the symptoms would pass and I would recover enough to at least go home and rest. My husband arrived almost immediately, and we talked through what had happened. I decided I just wanted to go home and rest it off. As he drove me home, I collapsed my head on the window and fell asleep, occasionally waking to ask him where we were. When we arrived home, he helped me make the journey to my bed. I was not as dizzy but felt as though someone had drugged me with a bear tranquilizer. My husband called my neurologist to inform him of what had happened, and to my lament, they advised us to go to the hospital. My stubbornness kicked in again; I told my husband I wanted to take a nap instead. (It is a shared assertion to say nurses are the worst patients.)

I spent the next 10 days in bed, in and out of deep sleep and semi-alert state. I only got up to use the bathroom and shower every couple of days. My appetite was non-existent, and I just wanted to sleep. Every time I tried to get up to do anything, it was as if my system powered down and did not allow me to do anything more than lie in bed. This was the hiatal crest of a four-month on/off migraine and the most intense season of stress I have ever experienced. Deep inside, I knew why this was happening. I had been operating on overdrive for months, if not years. I overworked, studied, exercised, and went from one commitment to the next without a narrow bathroom break in between. I was under such incredible stress that this level had become my standard operating procedure. I spent many nights crying myself to sleep because even though I had allowed these circumstances and made the choices to overload my plate; I didn't think it would have affected me in this way. I was an overachiever in anything that came across my radar. After this nervous system shut down, my neurologist shared that I likely had another episode of sterile brain inflammation (of which I had experienced once before in 2013, during the onset of hemiplegic migraines). He recommended I avoid any forms of extreme stimulation, to spend most of my time recuperating in bed for at least 14 days, and suggested I avoid the stimulating light of television and cell phones.

I had plenty of time to re-evaluate the state of my health during the three-week bedrest that followed. Not just my physical health expressed as neurological shutdown, but my relational, spiritual, emotional, mental, and occupational health was under duress. I knew this was the biggest wake-up call I needed to stop what I was doing. Looking back, my brain and body (namely, my hypothalamus, amygdala, and sympathetic nervous system) had been warning me for years. After exhausting all measures to restore homeostasis, my systems had finally given in and *shut down*. I later learned this was a system shut down because of an overworked and hyper reactive nervous system. It took me about four months to recover fully from that episode. Every time I thought I was feeling better, I would attempt a workout, try to clean the house, or even just go for a walk and my body said, "Nope. Not today, Elizabeth," and back to bed I went. Most days I had to spread out a 20-minute task over four to six hours, as not to cause my system to overreact.

An absence of balance supports disorder.

I share my story as a demonstration of what chronic stress can do to the nervous system. Not only was my nervous system chronically overstimulated, but I had also burned out my adrenal glands by pumping out inappropriate amounts of cortisol (the stress hormone). As previously noted, the hypothalamus receives information, interprets the information, and decides on an action that would best restore balance. Over time, a chronically anesthetized hypothalamus, insula, immune system, adrenal glands, and other neuroendocrine systems become depleted and stop working efficiently.

To emphasize how the brain responds to emotions and stressful events, the **insula** manages *reflective* emotions (such as responding to devastating news), whereas the **amygdala** responds with *automatic* emotions based on previous experiences (especially fear and trauma).

These two intricate areas translate physical experiences into emotions, and vice versa. In other words, *the body habitually follows the mind.* In a chronically overstressed migraine-prone brain, the processing of emotions may be distorted because of dysfunction in the insula. Thus, our body responds to our emotional state. We will explore more in depth how to break the stress response cycle in the chapter, *Stress and Emotions.* But first, let's examine the electrical system of the brain and body, and how to renovate this pathway to stop migraine attacks.

Chapter Three

The Electrical System and Faulty Wiring

He that wrestles with us strengthens our nerves and sharpens our skill.

Our antagonist is our helper.

-Edmund Burke

NOW THAT WE HAVE UNCOVERED THE SCIENCE behind migraines, you may be realizing that migraines hold far more complexity than they are often given credit for. Either that, or you are perplexed as to why I have dedicated all these pages to explaining intricate medical concepts. You would be justified in feeling that way, but here's the thing: many migraineurs are told that their migraines are simply exaggerated, prolonged headaches. Perhaps you have been told it yourself. This only causes frustration and confusion, as migraines truly are debilitating - so to be told that there is no clear root cause, no clear treatment, is disheartening at best. By breaking down the mechanisms behind migraines, you may be able to put a finger on what might be causing or worsening your suffering; further validating your pain experience in the context of your own personal life.

Let's now dig even deeper into migraine science - specifically, the electrical system of the migraine brain. Within the nervous system, we have a subsystem that operates automatically without conscious thought. This system, referred to as the **autonomic nervous system** (ANS), receives and processes information to elicit changes in our heart rate, blood pressure, breathing, pain perception, digestion, metabolism, and elimination. The ANS is further broken down into two opposing systems: the **sympathetic nervous system** (SNS), and the **parasympathetic nervous system** (PNS). Autonomic nervous system dysfunction and impaired function of the hypothalamus are well-documented in those who suffer from migraines. If you want to reveal how linked areas of the body function, short-circuit or disrupt one of them, and a disorder will emerge. Research has shown when strokes occur in the insula, it results in an increased chance of simultaneous dysfunction in the electrical system of the heart, such as an irregular heart rhythm. (Meyer et al., as cited by Borsook, 2016).

Disequilibrium of the two branches of the autonomic nervous system is clear, especially in the brains of migraineurs. The sympathetic nervous system is more commonly known as the "fight or flight" nervous system. When operating properly, this hyperarousal system prepares the body for immediate combat or running away from a threat or danger. Through a surge of hormones and glucose, the sympathetic nervous system is beneficial when a bear comes around the corner while you are hiking. However, when this system is chronically overstimulated, it is not so helpful in everyday life. The nervous system does not know the difference between the stress of a bear chasing you, versus stress from relationship strain, financial burdens, or chronic tension in the workplace. The brain perceives a threat and responds with swift reactions necessary to elicit action. Over time, this part of the nervous system becomes frayed and burned out, resembling Grandma's vacuum cleaner from 1964.

The sympathetic nervous system response is designed to keep humans safe from actual or perceived threats, such as from ravenous saber-toothed tigers while early humans foraged for berries. In modern days, the stress nervous system is helpful when we need to act quickly, such as to avoid hitting a car in front of us that slams on their brakes too quickly. We get that adrenaline jolt, our eyes widen, breath becomes rapid and shallow, and our reaction time becomes sharper. Afterwards, when the threat of safety has passed, we may still have tense muscles, be nauseated, and perhaps have a residual rapid heart rate. This response is expected in times of acute stress to get us through the event safely with maximum resources.

What about chronic, repeated, and long-standing stress? When a person lives regularly in the "fight or flight" mode, you can see how living in this state would eventually be detrimental to health and wellbeing. Faced with perceived stress, the sympathetic nervous system urgently evokes repeated fluctuations in various systems of the body to prepare for a fight or flight. Among these changes are:

- Increased heart rate, force of contraction, and electrical activity of the heart
- More airflow in lungs for increased oxygen delivery to muscles

- Decreased movement in the stomach and intestines to slow digestion, to shunt blood to the heart and lungs
- Decreased digestive and pancreatic enzymes
- Relaxation of the bladder and contraction of the sphincter to stop urine output
- Dilation of the eyes to allow more light to illuminate the environment
- Adrenal glands release norepinephrine (adrenaline) for immediate energy use, resembling a jolt from caffeine
- Glucose released from the liver to provide rapid energy throughout the body
- Apocrine sweat glands activate to increase sweating (perhaps this was an early genetic tactic to scare off a predator with offensive body odor)

So, what is the connection between the sympathetic nervous system and migraines? Since research shows stress to be the number one trigger for migraine, one theory is that chronic stress and over activation of the stress nervous system leads to depleted stores of norepinephrine and increased stores of inflammatory molecules such as prostaglandins and cytokines (known as adrenal burnout). An overtaxed sympathetic nervous system may lead to an excessive stress response in inappropriate situations. For example, two clients shared with me concerns they had about how they feel when they are under stress. "Why is it that every time I get bad news or am super stressed, I become nauseated and then it lasts for hours, sometimes days?" Another client said, "Every time I walk in to work and see my boss (who is making the demands of my job more stressful), I can feel my heart beating faster and I break out in hives." These are examples of **conditioned responses** of the sympathetic nervous system, when the brain prematurely and automatically responds to the stressor. In comparison to the Pavlovian Theory of a stimulus and reactive automatic response, the SNS then interprets these stressors as "get out or fight back" and over time, this system becomes hyperexcitable. I will discuss more about training the brain not to hyper respond to stress and how to cut down stress-induced migraines in the chapter, *Stress and Emotions.*

Migraines may result from chronic sympathetic nervous system overdrive, or because of an underactive **parasympathetic nervous system (PNS)**. We also know the parasympathetic nervous system as the "rest and digest" or "feed and breed" system (proposing that this system helps us stay calm, digest our food, and procreate). The true magic to achieving a state of balance and mitigating the incidence of migraine lies in this underutilized system. The PNS works to conserve energy by slowing the heart rate and breathing rate, constricting the pupils, producing tears, secreting saliva to help digest food, inhibiting adrenaline, allowing erections to occur, and relaxing nerves in the bladder. One measure of a well-conditioned PNS is a low resting heart rate (RHR). Healthy resting heart rates (the average heart rate per minute of a person at rest) should be between 60 and 100 beats per minute, and even as low as 40-50 in conditioned athletes. Conversely, the higher the resting heart rate, the higher the risk of health conditions. In the Copenhagen Male Study, researchers found that a resting heart rate between 81 and 90 doubles a person's risk of untimely death, while a RHR above 90 tripled the risk of premature death (Jensen, 2013). Therefore, a well-functioning parasympathetic nervous system keeps the body relaxed, and even lowers early cardiovascular death risk. The PNS plays a critical role in migraines, inflammation, and the sensation of pain since 75% of the parasympathetic nerve fibers come from the vagus nerve.

The Vagus Nerve

We can train the nervous system to stay calm and not overreact via a sweet spot called the **vagus nerve**, also known as the tenth cranial nerve. This wandering nerve is the longest cranial nerve in the body, exiting the brain stem (specifically the medulla oblongata) to travel a vagabond path into the outer covering of the brain, outer ear, carotid arteries, along the roof of the mouth, down the neck and through the larynx, through the esophagus, heart, lungs, and gut. The vagus nerve gives electrical rise to all organs from the neck down except the adrenal glands. The right branch of the vagus nerve controls the **sinoatrial (SA) node** of the heart, which acts as the pacemaker of the atria (upper chambers) of the heart. The left branch of the vagus nerve sends impulses to the **atrioventricular (AV) node**, starting further contraction of the ventricles (lower chambers) of the heart.

Here, anecdotal meets empirical. When I have experienced a migraine because of lack of sleep, nearly 99% of the time I would experience heart palpitations and an irregular heart rate. I recall sharing this finding with my former neurologist; he would say, "I have not heard of any correlation between migraine and heart palpitations." I would go home feeling defeated, knowing deep within my experience that there had to be a relationship between the two.

Let's peel apart the *why*. Whilst I have not conducted a study establishing a direct connection between migraines and heart palpitations, I did experience irregular and rapid rhythms of my heart when I developed a migraine related to sleep deprivation. When I was under extreme amounts of stress (which often would lead to lack of sleep), I can draw a personal hypothesis that perhaps the stress and lack of sleep sparked an overstimulated sympathetic nervous system, and a theoretically underactive parasympathetic nervous system by the way of faulty wiring impulses, leading to irregular and rapid resting heart rates.

The vagus nerve is also responsible for the *lowering* of the heart rate. When the vagus nerve is smoothly functioning in a state referred to as **vagal tone**, the nervous system is optimized in a state of calm, with clear and appropriate electrical messaging. Prior to the 1920s, it was unclear if signaling for the heart by the autonomic nervous system occurred through electrical impulses alone, or if biochemicals influenced the conductivity of the vagus nerve. It was through the work of German scientist Otto Loewi that a substance called **vagusstoff** was discovered. In one of his earliest studies, he extracted this liquid substance from a frog's electrically stimulated slow beating heart. Loewi then took vagusstoff liquid and applied it to another frog's heart that was beating fast. The application of vagusstoff made the second heart beat slower, showing the function of this biochemical liquid released by the vagus nerve. This research of vagusstoff birthed the discovery of the neurotransmitter, **acetylcholine**, which is released from the end terminals of the vagus nerve during deep, slow, mindful diaphragmatic exhalation. This tranquilizing and calming nectar counteracts the stimulating effects of norepinephrine (adrenaline) released by the sympathetic nervous system. To illustrate these two systems:

→ Stress or perceived threat
→ Sympathetic Nervous System activated
→ Norepinephrine (**adrenaline**) released
  → Increased heart rate and shallow, rapid breathing
  → Brain senses inflammation (**TNF-*a*, cytokines**) which causes a release of stress hormones to decrease inflammation (**cortisol**)

||

→ Deep, deliberate, diaphragmatic breathing with extended exhalation
  → Parasympathetic Nervous System activated (brain receives message that all is well)
  → Vagusstoff (acetylcholine) released
    → Heart rate slows, breathing slows
    → Sense of calm, homeostasis restored
    → Vagus nerve conditioned and toned

Remarkably, we can influence the responsiveness of the vagus nerve and keep the neural highway smooth by changing the information we give the nervous system. These are tangible examples of how we can change the course of the stress response in our bodies, by encouraging parasympathetic (rest) activation and decreasing over-reactivity of the sympathetic (stress) nervous system. The PNS and SNS serve as couriers between our immune, neurological, and **endocrine** (hormone) systems. In the next section of this book, I will reveal to you the methods to tone the vagus nerve and dilute an overcharged stress response, which can help you palliate stress-induced migraines.

*Author's note: I must mention that there can be too much of a good thing, as over-activation of the rest and digest mechanism can cause an extremely rare phenomenon called a vasovagal response, where brief loss of consciousness can occur. This response can occur during rapid lowering of the blood pressure due to sudden emotional stress, seeing blood, extreme coughing fits, straining to use the bathroom, lifting a heavyweight, or prolonged standing. In these rare occurrences, the vagus nerve is rapidly stimulated, causing a sudden drop in heart rate and blood pressure. Please note the keywords: **sudden and rapid**. It is remarkably unlikely that a vasovagal response would occur because of controlled, methodical, diaphragmatic breathing.*

SECTION TWO

THE METHODS TO RETRAIN THE BRAIN

Chapter Four

Sleep

Innocent sleep. Sleep that soothes away all our worries. Sleep that puts each day to rest. Sleep that relieves the weary laborer and heals hurt[ing] minds. Sleep, the main course in life's feast, and the most nourishing.

-William Shakespeare, *Macbeth*

"I CAN'T SLEEP." How many times have you said this, lying completely exhausted in your bed and yet unable to slip beneath the waves of slumber; rolling out of bed the next day just to stumble through your work or school tasks, barely keeping your eyes open? Or perhaps you are one of the thousands of people who suffer from frustrating 2 a.m. awakenings and have trouble getting back to sleep. You may feel that you are sleeping adequately, but perhaps still struggle with daytime fatigue, rarely feeling rested after a night of sleep.

I would speculate that, for migraineurs suffering from insufficient sleep, we have associated our sleeping room with enervating pain, undesirable feelings, suffering, and arduous self-warfare – all things that oppose calm, restorative sleep. Think about where you have spent most of your migraine recovery days. Likely, they were spent lying in that same bed where you are now trying to enjoy a relaxing, renewing night of sleep.

Insomnia

We associate insomnia or decreased sleep quality with a decrease in perceived health, because frankly, poor quality sleep makes us feel like garbage. I remember the exhausting years I spent sleeping less than four hours per night, suffocating beneath the jumbled mess I called my health. After my father died, the next six months I found myself 40 pounds overweight, overly stressed, and battling through 15-20 migraines a month. I mostly ate sweets and heavy carbohydrates, seeking comfort. I suffered from severe depression and was a zombie at work. My relationships were a shipwreck because I could not even focus long enough to care for myself. I look back now, relieved to have departed from that phase of my life, and wonder how regular, quality sleep could have balanced much of my overall health and well-being.

Insomnia is irrefutably connected to a host of poor outcomes. Those who suffer from it will often experience:

- decreased quality of life,
- increased perception of pain,
- frequent acute illnesses such as colds and infections,
- increased healthcare costs,
- and a heightened risk of injury.

Lack of habitual and restorative sleep can also lead to chronic conditions such as obesity, depression, heart disease, high blood pressure, diabetes, worsening migraine frequency, and aggravation of chronic pain. Additionally, poor sleep has been linked to an increased risk of Alzheimer's disease. Sleep is essential to anyone seeking a life without the burden of disease - and certainly to those trying to free themselves of migraines. Lack of sleep permits an increase of proteins in the brain that are known to trigger inflammation and the pain response, leading to the homeostasis domino effect we know precipitates a migraine. On the flip side, taking a Saturday morning snooze-in to "catch up" on lost sleep may seem like a great idea to restore lost sleep, however it is a disruption to your sleep pattern. Oversleeping, napping too frequently, or any other disruption to your normal sleep pattern can also produce migraines.

For your brain to function optimally, it is critical that you are going to bed and waking up at nearly the same time, every day, seven days a week. The brain craves consistency. In this chapter, I will share with you not only how to improve the quality of your sleep, but how to prioritize sleep to reduce migraine occurrence. But first, let's explore what happens in the brain and body as we sleep.

Understanding sleep

Sleep is more than just lying still with our eyes closed. Instead, it is a very active process, and one that is necessary for life. It is a time where the brain plays an active role in restoring hormones, repairing body tissues, and consolidating memories and newly learned information. When we give our brains the necessary estimated 33% of our day to be in a state of sleep, these functions can take place organically. If we deprive the brain of this critical restorative time, messages are sent to the nervous system that there is an imbalance. Think of sleep as the recalibration of our entire day. When it cannot recalibrate and restore, this precipitates dysfunction in the brain's insula, leading to poor decision making and altered control over bodily functions. A disruption in appetite hormones can inspire overeating, specifically of junk foods that are high in fat, sugar, and carbohydrates, thus inviting a whole other host of issues.

We can seriously disrupt our hormones with continual sleep deprivation, to the point of precipitating disease or disorder. For instance, chronic lack of sleep is associated with insulin resistance and increased blood sugars. To a person with diabetes, this can cause their disease to worsen. Chronic sleep deprivation can also prompt disease in someone who was previously unaffected. Further, a lack of sex drive has been linked to sleep deprivation, since a minimum of three hours of uninterrupted sleep is needed for testosterone production to occur. Other mood-related conditions such as depression and anxiety can be similarly activated or worsened by chronic sleep deprivation. The immune system and blood pressure are also put at risk. Considering that this is in no way an exhaustive list of the possible harmful effects of poor sleep, evidently, sleep is critically linked to wellbeing.

We often take sleep for granted and push it to the bottom of our priority list. When I am working with new clients, this is the first topic we approach together. Sleep must be the first step in working toward a migraine-free life.

The Circadian Rhythm

High-quality restorative sleep cleans out the cobwebs of the brain, which restores clarity, a balanced mood, and lowers levels inflammation. Ideally, we should spend a third of our life asleep. Take one-third of your current age - that's a substantial portion. With sleep such an essential part of life, there must be an orderly sequence for sleep to be effective. We refer to this sequence of events that occurs ritually as a **circadian rhythm**. Circadian rhythms are occurring every 24 hours, yearly, and with a rhythmic seasonal cycle. So then, what prompts sleep to occur? Our brain picks up on cues from the environment that signal the brain to prepare for sleep. Each of these cues is referred to as a **zeitgeber,** which synchronizes the biological rhythm to the earth's 24 hours and 12-month light/dark cycle. These cues include sunlight exposure, exercise, temperature, social interactions, routine, and eating.

Sunlight and blue light are the strongest zeitgebers. Even when our eyes are closed, photoreceptors in the eyes can still light, which inhibits preparation for sleep and tells our brain to "stay awake." Sound familiar? You have probably experienced something like this before. Perhaps you've come home from an exhausting day at work – and become groggy at around 7-8 p.m., accidentally falling asleep on the couch. Then, after waking up to go to bed, you lie scrolling through social media or the latest news articles on your phone. You glare into your bright screen and say to yourself, "I just can't fall asleep!" Light, especially the blue light emitted from electronic devices such as phones, tablets, and televisions, tells the **pineal gland** in the brain *not* to release melatonin. The normal daily release of melatonin is around 8-9 p.m. - we release it according to the cues given in the circadian rhythm. If this release is disrupted, our brains struggle to prepare us properly for sleep. (More on melatonin in the chapter, *Hormones and Biochemicals*.)

We should spend one-third of our life asleep.

Appetite and Sleep

Do you ever notice that your appetite increases after a night or two of not enough sleep? Or, if you are a shift worker, do you notice that you are prone to snack all night while at work, then return home to sleep for a few hours, then wake up and eat again? Lack of quality sleep (or working during evening or night shifts) disrupts normal sleep circadian rhythms and alters appetite hormone levels. This can lead to excessive sleepiness, decreased energy, trouble concentrating, headaches, migraines, and mood changes, especially irritability. It is estimated that even one night of poor sleep makes the amygdala 60% more reactive, which is why you might be more short-tempered with your coworkers or family the next day.

Long-term shift work can also lead to obesity, depression, high blood pressure, chronic inflammation and, in the migraineur, a pull toward more medication for migraine management. The root of excessive cravings related to poor sleep has to do with two appetite hormones that are normally regulated while we sleep. I will explain these hormones more in Chapter Six, and how to reduce cravings through gut health.

Sleep Cycles, Stages, and Brain Waves

Just as seasons of nature follow a cycle, so do our brains. The brain prefers rhythmic consistency to stay high functioning. One of the ways we can measure the brain's cyclical functions is through brain waves. Similar to musical notes, **brain waves** are electrical impulses sent between neurons. These electrical impulses vary at different times throughout a 24-hour period and can be affected by the rate and depth of the breath, stress, sleep, medications, and disease processes such as epilepsy or migraines. **Low frequency** brain waves are like the deep beat of a drum or bassoon, whereas **high frequency** brain waves are like that of a whistle or piccolo. When brain waves are slow, we are sleepy, dreamy, relaxed, and calm. When brain waves are high pitched and quick, we are hyper aroused, or alert and wired.

Sleep cycles and **stages of sleep** are vitally important to measure the quality and restorative function of sleep. We can compare cycles and stages of sleep to washing clothes. For each complete load of laundry (each load equals a sleep cycle), it first starts with putting the clothes in, shutting the lid, and filling the washing basin (stage one of sleep), then a gentle swirl to wet the clothes (stage two), then the soap permeates the fabrics and wash away dirt and stains (stages three and four), and then the final rinse and spin (stage five). Now the question I must pose rhetorically is, would you ever stop the wash cycle midway, grab the drenched clothes, and wear them to work? Of course, you would not - the soaked, half-washed clothes would cause a world of discomfort.

As it happens, we essentially do this to ourselves when we interrupt our sleep cycles. Instead of soggy clothes, however, we are faced with intense grogginess upon awakening; we hit the snooze button repeatedly, then finally get up, stumbling through the day in an irritable fog. Some may view this as a small price to pay for a flexible sleep schedule. For migraineurs, however, an inconsistent sleep pattern can mean a self-induced migraine attack, no longer a minor inconvenience, but a significant and painful strain on the day. Steady sleep patterns are essential to a migraineur's journey of recovery. I will share with you how to stop interrupting your natural sleep rhythm – and how to feel rested and alert, to sustain energy, and to avoid unnecessary migraine attacks.

Let's first gain a better understanding of the sleep cycles and stages. A complete sleep cycle is the process of completing the five stages of sleep, just as a washing machine goes from rinse, to wash, to spin, and so forth. In one complete sleep cycle, there are five vital stages the brain must go through. You may have heard of **REM** (rapid eye movement) sleep mentioned before; this is one of the stages, along with **NREM** (non-rapid eye movement) light sleep and NREM deep sleep. The stages do not progress in a linear fashion, as one might think. They skip back and forth dynamically, starting with NREM light sleep, then moving to NREM deep sleep, then reversing back to light sleep, then onward to REM sleep. Once a cycle is complete, another begins. For optimal restorative sleep, four-to-six complete cycles (lasting around 90-minutes each) is the sweet spot. This is where the general six-to-nine-hour sleep recommendation originates.

Have you ever had the 'falling dream'? The one where, right as you fall asleep, you feel a sensation of plummeting through the air uncontrollably; your muscles jerk, panicked, and you wake up just before you hit the bottom? This likely sounds familiar, as it is an experience shared by many people upon entering the **first stage of sleep**. This stage is called **light NREM**, in which your body is preparing to succumb to a vulnerable state. Think of the first stage starting after arranging the sleeping space, putting on pajamas, lying the head down on the pillow, pulling the blankets up, and aligning the body into the most comfortable position. Light NREM helps prepare the brain, mind, and body for deep sleep. During this time, we are in a conscious early sleep state, lasting anywhere from one to seven minutes. We can awaken from this point and feel as though we did not sleep at all.

In stage one of sleep, the brain is exhibiting **alpha** and **theta** waves. Alpha waves, the power of the present, are where relaxed mindfulness and awareness take place. Theta waves follow as we fall asleep to enhance memory, learning, and intuition. These theta waves allow us to focus our consciousness inward, tuning out the external world. They are also the frequency of brain waves where we hold our subconscious fears.

As we progress to stage two, brain waves calm down, the heart rate slows, and body temperature drops. This is the stage of power naps; the first segment of **deep NREM** sleep, where brain waves are sending small bursts of activity called spindles and K-complexes. This activity helps to stay asleep and prevents accidental awakening. Stage two lasts approximately 20 minutes.

The bread and butter of recuperative sleep is contained within stages three and four. This is a time of deep, subconscious activity where there is no eye movement, minimal muscle activity, and a very low chance of awakening. When you are not sleeping well, you may tend to have less energy, experience more pain, or be more prone to illness. This is because during NREM stages three and four, the immune system is boosted, muscle and tissue injuries are all being repaired, and hormones are restored and released. This stage of repair and recovery is often overlooked, yet it facilitates the critical act of restoring energy at the cellular level. Brain waves during these stages resemble a loud and low drumbeat, as **delta** waves permeate our entire system, encouraging suspension of external awareness and dreamless sleep.

The last stage of sleep in a complete cycle is stage five, **REM sleep**. In REM sleep, the brain is most active; the eyes dart back and forth, the muscles are paralyzed (except the heart and diaphragm), and the heart rate and blood pressure elevate. Breathing is rapid and shallow, and will often mimic the sleeping person's dream activity, as this is the stage in which most dreaming occurs. Brain waves during REM are rapid and erratic, like the frequencies of alertness. This is when coagulated learning is solidified and memories are stored. In your waking life, if you find yourself walking into a room and forgetting why you entered in the first place (or other examples of short-term memory loss), it may be due to disrupted REM sleep. A high-quality sleeper will experience five to six REM cycles per night; and as the night progresses (if sleep is uninterrupted), each REM cycle gets longer, with the last REM cycle lasting up to one hour. However, the frequency and duration of REM sleep *decreases* with age.

Waking up in the middle of stages three, four, or five may leave one feeling disoriented, groggy, moody, and particularly unrested. This grogginess is referred to as **sleep inertia**, or **Hicham's Syndrome,** and is most likely to occur if awoken during stage three of sleep. It leaves the sleeper stuck in a precarious state between waking and sleeping where the body desires to sleep deeply but is unable to. The best way to avoid sleep inertia is to wake up either naturally without an alarm, or at the end of a sleep cycle. So, when you set your alarm for 6:15 a.m. every morning, how do you know what stage you are waking up in? Do you notice that some mornings you feel rested, and other mornings you feel groggy and disoriented? Allow me to share with you how you can wake up at the end of a sleep cycle and feel alert and rested for optimized health with the first step of *The Migraine Method.*

Method #1: Train Your Brain to Sleep

Many people, especially those with migraines, may pragmatically say, "I know I could sleep better, but honestly I think I am sleeping fine." Or, they may pessimistically say, "I have tried it all - you name it. I cannot sleep. My brain doesn't shut off, and I just lay there." You might have found yourself in one of these two categories, or curious about how to sleep better. We are about to explore how you can improve your sleep to balance hormones, appetite, weight, *and* migraine occurrence - so grab a pen, and let's get started.

To work this step, I encourage you to commit to at least six to seven days per week of consistency. Within two to three weeks, you should be able to train your brain to respond well to sleep cues, reaping the incredible benefits of revitalizing sleep. The methods for restoring your sleep to reduce migraine occurrence are what I call Therapeutic Improvements to Promote Sleep (TIPS).

» If you drink caffeine, finish your last caffeinated beverage before 2 p.m.

Caffeine is a known stimulant. It can disrupt normal sleep cycles, reducing your overall duration and depth of sleep. Caffeine also has a long half-life, which means your cup of joe takes longer to clear out of your system than you think.

If you drink 200 mg of a caffeinated beverage at 8 a.m., at 2 p.m. there will still be 100 mg in your system. In that case, drinking a cup of coffee at 2 p.m. will leave you with at least half of that caffeine in your system at bedtime. Be mindful of how much caffeine you are drinking throughout the day, as it has a cumulative effect on the brain. Caffeine and alcohol disrupt sleep cycles and decrease the likelihood to get into a deep REM cycle. Consuming these substances near bedtime can interrupt sleep cycles and lead to the proverbial 2 a.m. awakening (more on alcohol in the chapter on *Nutrition and Gut Health*).

» No light past 8 p.m.

The light-sensitive neurotransmitter **melatonin** naturally releases between 8 and 9 p.m. As you start your wind down for the evening, set an alarm reminding yourself to avoid artificial light from phones, TVs, laptops, or tablets beyond 8-9 p.m. Lamps with red light are conducive to sleep, so if you choose, you may replace a bulb with a red light or incandescent bulb in the bedroom. Avoid LED, fluorescent, or halogen bulbs, as these emit blue light that stimulates the brain. (It may be of importance to note that these types of lights should be avoided by migraineurs at all times, as they can increases neuro-sensitivity.)

» Determine your sleep and wake time based on sleep cycles.

For peak health, four to six sleep cycles per night is an ideal number to strive for. There are a few ways to make sure you are waking up at the end of a sleep cycle. First, if your schedule does not warrant setting a morning alarm, allow your body to wake up naturally in the morning. The first time you awaken, if it has been at least six hours, *stay awake.* Your brain will generally wake you up after at least four cycles at the end of a completed cycle (akin to washing a load of laundry). If you require an alarm to get up at the same time every morning, you will do the reverse by counting backwards by 90-minute cycles to know what time to go to bed.

The easiest way to calculate what time to go to bed or to rise is to use an app such as **Sleepyti.me** (see Resources in the back of this book). Enter the time you need to wake up, and the algorithm will determine what times to fall asleep to wake up at the end of a sleep cycle. For example: if I need to wake up at 5:15 a.m., the best times to fall asleep are 8:15 p.m., 9:45 p.m., 11:15 p.m., or 12:45 a.m. If you go to sleep outside of those times, you may possibly wake up groggy in a state of sleep inertia. If you are awake beyond 8:15 p.m., it is better to wait until the next recommended sleep time (in this example, 9:45 p.m.) to avoid sleep inertia. Write your wake time here _____, and your recommended sleep times here _____.

» Use a sleep cycle alarm clock.

If you must wake up at prescriptive times and would like to monitor your sleep quality even closer, I suggest using the app, **Sleep Cycle Alarm Clock** (see Resources). This app works on your phone (next to the bed but not in the bed) to monitor the sounds you make during sleep, such as rolling over, snoring, or heavy breathing. I have used this myself and for clients and find that it is accurate for waking up at the end of a sleep cycle. There are options to use a gentle awakening alarm, which is a 30-minute window prior to your exact wake-up time. This is helpful to wake you up prior to you going into another cycle of sleep. You can monitor your sleep quality percentages over time, showing trending in your sleep quality.

Keep in mind, cortisol (the stress hormone to energize you for your day) rises in the early morning hours, and peaks between 6 and 7 a.m., so it is best to wake up by then.

Author's Note: I do not recommend wearing an electronic watch to bed unless you have notifications turned off, so that they do not wake you.

» Start a Sleep Kit.

At the same time every night (within a 60-minute window), start your preparation for bed. Give yourself at least 45 minutes to prepare before you plan on falling asleep. In this sleep kit, you will include three to four items or practices that you will only do at bedtime.

For example, you might choose to:

- Use a certain facial cleanser or lavender-scented lotion as you prepare for bed - brush your teeth, brush your hair, and rub lotion on your feet
- Read a familiar poem out of the same book, or write in a gratitude journal
- Write a brief journal entry of anything that is bothering you, or a reminder for tomorrow so you don't lie awake thinking about your to-do list or obsessing over things you cannot control

If stress is bothering you or you feel anxious before bed, you may even want to write your feelings down on a slip of paper and *throw it away.*

This may symbolically help you release any emotions or thoughts that would impede on falling or staying asleep. Keep a small basket in your bathroom or on your nightstand that contains these items or rituals for your sleep kit. It is important to have the same routine every single night, regardless of your schedule the next day. After a few days of this practice, you may start to sense the secretion of melatonin, and become drowsy while completing your sleep routine.

» Listen to the same song or guided meditation every night.

As you work towards training the brain for high quality sleep, an auditory cue such as the same song every night will also help the brain associate that song with sleep. You may play this song as you are completing your bedtime routine or wait until you have laid down. Choose a song slow in tempo that you find relaxing. Instrumental songs are best, or guided meditations by the same person each night. Do not play this song or meditation at any other time besides bedtime.

» Use your bedroom only for sleep and sex.

It is so tempting to work from bed, watch T.V., or even do another brain stimulating activity such as emails, work, or homework. It is imperative that you use the bed you intend on sleeping in only for sleep and sexual activity. This will help the brain recognize the bed space for sleep and rest and not stay activated for higher processing activities.

» Wear an eye mask at night.

Since we know that the absence of light stimulates the pineal gland to release melatonin, a simple way to eliminate ambient light is to apply an eye mask over the eyes as you lie down. Keep in the sleep kit your eye mask, eye pillow, or even a small washcloth to cover the eyes.

» Destroy negative thoughts.

Self-talk such as "I will never fall asleep, this won't work... I am already not feeling well, so tomorrow will suck..." will tell the brain and body to respond according to exactly what you are saying. Remember, the *body follows the mind.* Infuse your thoughts and body with encouraging and relaxing thoughts, such as, "I am the best version of myself right now; I am prioritizing my health because I deserve to feel well. I have loved myself and loved others to the best of my ability today." Recall three things that you are sincerely grateful for right before sleep or imagine a person that you hold deep affection or appreciation for as you drift off to sleep.

» Go with the release.

Allow sleep to happen naturally, instead of "trying" to fall asleep. The more you think about falling asleep, the less naturally it may occur. As you continue to develop a regular sleep preparation practice, the easier it becomes and more quickly you will fall asleep. It is important to note, you may get out of bed if you are feeling restless beyond 15-20 minutes, so that your brain does not associate the bed with restlessness or anxiety. If this happens, return to your sleep kit and start again.

» Open headspace for body relaxation.

Good sleep starts during the day. If we wait until bedtime to clear the stress of the day, we may find ourselves prey to insomnia. Non-sleep deep rest (NSDR) is the protective covering and daytime stress clearing for the brain. This can be done by 15-30 minutes of meditation during the day, to charge up the parasympathetic nervous system (more on this in Chapter Ten). Some nights I find myself a little more restless than usual. On these nights, it is helpful to listen to guided meditations and practice a body scanning meditation to allow my mind and body to relax. If you listen to a guided meditation, find one that works for you and relaxes you. Make sure the voice and the music are relaxing and not annoying. My current favorite is by Jason Stephenson on YouTube. I have also recorded a special guided meditation for you on my website, www.elizabethpriller.com (see Resources).

» Practice focused breathing.

As you lie down, it is imperative to prepare the body for sleep. Start by lying down in a comfortable position, preferably on your back or side. Make sure every part of your body feels supported and the position you would like to fall asleep in. Start by taking a slow deep breath in through your nose, pause, and exhale slowly for four to six seconds. (Remember, the slow, intentional exhale helps release vagusstoff and activate relaxation). Continue to focus on your breath, on a slow inhale, and even slower exhale. Focus on your breathing in the diaphragm, or belly-breathing. Let the chest relax as you breathe. Allow your shoulders to drop away from the ears, relax your forehead, eyes, mouth, jaw, and arms. Release your tongue from the roof of the mouth and allow the lips to part slightly if that feels right for you. (More on breathing techniques in the chapter *Yoga, Meditation, and Breath).*

» Set a goal.

Besides the action steps, set a personal sleep goal. Make sure your goal is specific, measurable, attainable, realistic, and time sensitive. How do you want to feel when you lie down, and when you awaken?

Example goals are:
- I want to wake up rested at least four of seven nights of therapeutic sleep
- I will practice my sleep routine at least six out of seven nights for at least two weeks
- I will drink herbal tea versus caffeine tea after 2 p.m.
- I will choose and use at least three items for my sleep kit by the end of this week
- At least five of seven nights I will have sleep quality above 70% (if using the Sleep Cycle Alarm Clock)

- I will release any negative thought patterns before I go to bed by writing them down and replacing the thought with a positive thought, saying it three times.

Therapeutic Sleep Plan

What is your goal for this section about sleep?

What other positive actions will you take every day to encourage therapeutic sleep?

Go through each step of the sleep method and write down your individualized plan.

Chapter Five

Stress and Emotions

Every cell in your body is eavesdropping on your thoughts.

-Deepak Chopra

THE STRESS RESPONSE IN THE BODY presents itself in three stages: alert or alarm, resist or adapt, and exhaustion. When the threat of stress first comes into your emotional, mental, or physical space, the initial reaction of the brain is to sound the alarm. The alarm in the brain goes off to alert you that there is a threat, just like the smoke detector in your home, or a burglar alarm in a department store. The **alarm** stage may bring with it a racing heartbeat, nausea, stomachaches, backaches, headaches, changes in appetite, or difficulty sleeping. You can compare this stage to a smoke detector in your home; when the alarm goes off, it is signaling that something is wrong. It is then your job to take care of said problem (or call a professional) - the house cannot fix itself. Our bodies and minds are the same way. The alarm goes off, but it is our job to make adjustments to prevent further damage.

The next stage of stress response in the body is **resist or adapt**, and this is where further damage can form. Imagine a house fire, with fire and smoke rapidly expanding from the initial "alarm" to adjacent rooms in the house, setting off secondary alarms as it creates a path of destruction. In the body, though we may notice the first alarm of looming stress, we unfortunately condition ourselves to ignore this second alarm. We continue burning, figuratively and literally, neglecting ourselves and continuing lifestyle behaviors that cause further inflammation in the body. In doing so, we pave the way for damaging symptoms like headaches, stomach troubles, high blood pressure, or under/overeating. The body and brain can adapt to this stage for a short time, as compensatory mechanisms in the body will adjust to keep us alive past the alarm phase. As my friend put this counterintuitively, "I occasionally anxiously lean into life like I need to see the threat better." Long-term, however, this ignorance leads to the **exhaustion** phase, where the body and brain wave the white flag in surrender.

Imagine trying to breathe and work in a burning building for weeks-your wellbeing would deteriorate quickly. Therefore, disease or disorder form if we do not react to the alarms and fail to make changes. Eventually, the body and brain say, "No more". The fiery pathway to disease becomes a well-lit freeway. I can imagine our personified brains saying, "Well, I tried to warn you, but you didn't listen. I tried to hand you a fire extinguisher, but you ignored me. I tried to call on my other systems to help you, but they are exhausted now, too. So, if you want to sit in a burning house, you are on your own."

While this may be a harsh illustration of stress and its implications, this is our reality. Migraine sufferers are some of the most stubborn stress adapters (speaking from experience - I am no exception). We can be told to slow down, to take a break, to focus on ourselves, but we keep on pushing. When stress infiltrates our day, we allow it to consume us, propagating anxiety, anger, bitterness, and grief like a rapidly spreading fire. So, what do you notice about your migraine patterns? Can you expect an almost guaranteed avalanche of symptoms after you have had a fight with a loved one, or after a particularly stressful day at work? When you forget to eat breakfast and lunch? When are you holding tension in your body? When you exchange dinner for half a bottle of wine to "decompress"? How does your body feel when you are anxious, and your breathing is shallow and rapid? How does your body respond when you allow lack of forgiveness, lingering bitterness, or negative self-talk to become a part of everyday life?

While these questions may seem like accusatory or unpleasant inquiries, they are areas of my life that I had to appraise before I started to change my experience with migraines. I wish someone had asked me these questions, or that I had been bold enough to ask myself sooner. This kind of self-examination is confronting, and I recognize that you may not be ready for this level of intense vulnerability. I respect where you are right now. My hope is that this chapter will help you explore areas of your life where perhaps you had not identified a trigger for migraines before. After you identify these areas and implement methods in response, you can change your entire migraine experience.

Stress

Put simply, stress is any threat to homeostasis that prompts us to adapt or respond. Just as a bridge has a structural weight limit, we have a psychological and physical stress limit which determines our breaking point. Of course, the figurative "break" we see here comes in the form of migraines, stomach and intestinal disturbances, nausea, fatigue, or mood changes - all bodily responses to an excessive load of stress. Most of pain is buried in the central nervous system, and our emotional and psychological state further drives the pain experience. If our emotions are erratic and we feel we are *under* stress, we experience more pain. Changing the ways in which we react to stress will transform the way our brain and body respond to the perception of the pain threshold.

The migraine brain is a brain in conflict.

We can perceive stress as *actual, reactive,* or *anticipatory.* How many times do we worry or stress about something that has not occurred, only to find we stressed over it for nothing? For example, we may hear that a thunderstorm is brewing and proceed to stress about it all the way to work, even though the sun is shining with no storm clouds in sight. This is **anticipatory stress**. When we worry, we are sending messages to our brain and body to prepare for a fight or flight reaction. Toxic thought patterns such as ruminating, worrying, dwelling on anxious thoughts, or creating scenarios in our minds can release stress hormones. It is these hormones which flood the body with cortisol and adrenaline, pump sugar into the bloodstream, and potentially trigger a migraine attack. Simply thinking about a past stressful event can engage the autonomic nervous system re-engage the body for fight or flight.

Every time we think about a negative event from our past, our body produces the same chemicals it did when the event first took place. Psychologist and author Bessel van der Kolk wrote, "Trauma comes back as a reaction [in the body], not a memory." Every migraine attack can be categorically traumatic; we often remember the events, people, and activities we missed because of a migraine. In van der Kolk's book, *The Body Keeps Score*, he explores the mind's impact on the body in this sense. "In order to change, people need to realize their sensations and how their bodies interact with the world around them. Physical self-awareness is the first step in releasing the tyranny of the past." Part of conquering the migraine experience is discovering the connection between your mind and your body and creating a well-adjusted relationship between the two.

The migraine brain is a brain in conflict. Often associated with migraines are conditions such as depression, anxiety, and other mental health comorbidities. For me personally, a shift in my mood towards depression or anxiety would always accompany the onset of a migraine; once the migraine lifted, my mood would return to baseline. This relief was often temporary, however, as anxious feelings tended to creep back in post-migraine. Much like hearing a daunting weather forecast, my brain succumbed to anxiety in anticipation of the next migraine attack. Anticipatory anxiety floods the body with the same emotions as anxiety in the present - if you have ever felt anxious in the absence of a migraine, your brain may be fearing an attack that has not yet arrived.

Disordered mood processing occurs due to changes in the limbic system, the insula, and the hypothalamus. The **limbic system** is home to some of our most integral mental departments: the **amygdala**, where we process fear; the **hippocampus**, where our memories are stored; and the **hypothalamus**, where homeostasis is regulated. Emotions are regulated by the limbic system. Consider this part of the brain our personal security guard and historian, creating and storing the emotion securely with the memory. For example - think about the smell of crayons, the name of your favorite teacher, or the playground you spent hours playing on in elementary school. If I were to ask you to tell me about these memories, what emotions would accompany them? When you reflect upon your childhood, how often do you become lost in the nostalgic flurry of emotions that come back as you reminisce? The same is true of memories that hold anger, sadness, grief, or anxiety. For example, revisiting an old workplace where you experienced an emotional, mental, or physical trauma would bring back some of the uncomfortable emotions you experienced while working there.

Memories and emotions are bound by the limbic system acting as our emotional archive – with our sensations bound to the events. Our migraine experiences are no exception to this. As a migraineur, you can probably recall places or events where migraines have incapacitated your well-being and your capacity to enjoy life; the places you have had to lie down because of nausea or dizziness, or the times where you have had to leave a social gathering half-way through; or the fights you have had with loved ones after migraines ruthlessly infiltrated your relationships. The reason short-term experiences are stored into long-term memories is because a significant emotion is tied to that memory. In migraineurs, often this process is faulty, leading to a cycle of hyper-interpretation of stressors, memories, or environmental stimuli.

The HPA Axis and Migraines

As the pressures of mental, emotional, or physical stress invade the body, a specific network in the brain is responsible for releasing stress hormones: the **HPA (hypothalamus-pituitary-adrenal) axis**. Beyond just the hypothalamus, the HPA axis is an interconnected system that correlates emotions, stress, and hormones. This hub is awakened by anticipatory stress or actual stress; and once activated, it releases a flood of stress hormones from the adrenal glands. These stress hormones are again an attempt to meet the energy demands imposed on our body. Over time, chronic stress can lead to exhaustion of the adrenal glands, obesity, diabetes, high blood pressure, and cyclic migraine occurrence.

There are many factors that influence an individual's response to **acute** (sudden) or **chronic** (long-term and repeated) physical or psychological stress. Factors such as genetics, prior life experiences in the family unit, environmental exposures, age, and sex can affect how one handles stress. For example, women tend to have more HPA axis activation with psychological stress than men. How individuals handle stress (both in the acute and chronic stages) determines whether the stress responses are *adaptive* or *maladaptive*. Maladaptive stress responses can lead to disease or disorder, such as chronic migraines.

Chronic stress deprives us of an appropriate response for a life-threatening event.

The system we have for responding to stress is a critical and highly effective one, designed to boost our energy and physical ability when faced with a life-threatening stressor. It is important to remember, however, that cumulative chronic stress can render our stress response system dangerous, malfunctional, or ineffective altogether; if our HPA axis is overstimulated, the adrenal glands become desensitized, and cortisol levels are more difficult to regulate. Think about a doorbell that gets pushed once per month, versus a doorbell that rings every day at 5 a.m., 7:30 a.m., 8:15 a.m., 11:10 a.m., 12:14 p.m., 1:44 p.m., 3:10 p.m., 5:33 p.m., etc. Which doorbell do you think will last longer? If you had to hear each of those doorbells, which one would you tune out after the third, fourth, or fifth push? Comparative is our nervous system's response to chronic stress. After those first few doorbell rings (stressors), the nervous system will be on hyper-alert. If the doorbell rings repetitively, however, the nervous system will eventually tune out the stressors and produce erratic responses. It almost sounds good on paper- having your body stop responding to stress – as a racing heart and squeamish stomach are not pleasant reactions by any means. Unfortunately, however, profound chronic stress and an insufficient response of the HPA axis will deprive the individual of an *appropriate* response to a life-threatening event. At various points in our lives, we will be faced with circumstances where we need an increased flow of oxygen to our lungs, more adrenaline coursing through our veins, and more energy being pumped through our body. However, if the nervous system has been run down by chronic stress, those important responses will struggle to take place when we need them most. Not only does chronic stress weaken the responses, but it also generates a surplus of cortisol. This leads to a host of inflammatory health issues – and most notably in the vein of this book, migraines.

Long-term cortisol release beyond the daily morning dose can lead to increased levels of inflammatory chemical messengers called cytokines and prostaglandins, such as IL-6 and TNF-*a*. We already know that TNF-*a* is associated with the onset of a migraine, which can trigger the trigeminal nerve and subsequently stimulate the release of CGRP. As we uncover the cascading events that trigger a migraine, we can see loopholes of how to stop a migraine in its tracks; as many of these biological events are the targeted areas of drug treatments for migraines (though, these drugs are not without unpleasant side effects). Just as if the check engine light of our car were to light up, we would suspect an issue with the car's operation. Our bodies are no different. A migraine is just one of the many warning signs of unmanaged chronic stress.

A mind in an overwhelmed state
can mobilize stress in the whole body.

Let me share a story about the perception of stress. After a particularly hectic week at work, I went for my first facial at a local spa. As I walked into a calm, dimly lit room, where another patron, Lucy, and I were greeted by the estheticians. We were asked simple questions: "Is this your first facial? How would you describe your skin type?" Their last question was, "Are you under any stress?" To which I thought, *who is not under some form of stress?* Well, Lucy's answer caused me to spin my neck around like Regan from the 1970s thriller. She quaintly replied, "No." I could hardly believe what I was hearing. *Not under stress?* At the time, I was in grad school full-time, teaching 12-14 hours per day, had just moved to a new city, and was planning a wedding (I now look back on this time as a perfect Julia Child-esque recipe for Stress Souffle). For years after this encounter at the spa, my mind still could not come to grips with the idea of a life not strangled by stress.

Fast forward, after deep lifestyle changes and essential lessons learned the hard way, it makes sense to me. Think about the concept of being "under stress." When Lucy answered "no" to the estheticians, she was not implying that stress didn't exist in her life at all; instead that she was not *under it*. She was not *below stress, not being crushed by it, not barely breathing because of the weight of it*. Stress had probably been present in some form in her life, but either she had a well-greased valve to relieve the pressure, or she had a way of not allowing it to crush her. Considering this realization, I have changed the way I talk about and relate to stress. I no longer *have* stress, nor am I *under* stress. These terms represent possessive ways of holding the stress in our mind and body. Instead, I give powerful words to the stress experience, such as, "I do not know how I will handle the loss of my dog, and her death makes me feel sad. I can feel that sadness in my chest. I am choosing to acknowledge the sadness, but a stressful event will not define or control how I choose to respond."

We both know that even though facials can be enjoyable and relaxing, they are not likely to relieve all the pressures of work stress, raising kids, mowing the yard, fights with our loved ones, the furnace going out, more monthly expenses than money, world wars, health crises, social divides, and the other burdens we hold in a balancing act on our shoulders. These are the stressors that can infiltrate our headspace unchecked, overtaking the 1,700 centimeters^3 of the area in between our ears. With so much space at its disposal, is it any surprise that mental, emotional, relational, occupational, financial, physical, or spiritual stress can pre-curse pain in the head? Considering that the two hours after an outburst of anger can increase one's risk of a heart attack fivefold, we know that there is a deeply rooted connection between emotions and the physical body. If we don't acknowledge and address this, unraveled emotions can become a migraineur's worst enemy. So let's empower ourselves with method number two.

Method #2: Mitigate Your Reactivity to Stress

How do we realistically mitigate our stress response and balance our emotions when stress is still present? Rather than trying to eliminate the stress, we must learn to interact with stressful situations in a more level way. Emotions are *e-motion*, or energy in motion. Just as Newton's Third Law of Motion states, "every action has an equal and opposite reaction," every episode of perceived or actual stress lends an opportunity to elicit an equal reaction in the body. The way we connect with the stress determines somewhat of how our bodies respond. Sometimes we can function at a high level of stress for a period, but in due time, without a release, we will break. Let me share with you how to rewire the brain's way of responding to stress so that over time, you can rewire the stress response.

>> Identify where you feel stress.

Take your right hand and place it on the space of your body where you feel stress. When you get bad news, when you are anxious, when you are under stress, where do you feel it in your physical body? Where do you notice tension, pain, heat, nausea, strain, or discomfort? Chances are you placed your right hand on either your head, chest, or stomach - coincidentally, the path of the vagus nerve. We hear the cliché phrase, "Listen to your gut." Well, there is a science behind that statement, and we will explore that more in the chapter, *Nutrition and Gut Health*.

>> Identify what triggers your stress.

For the final six-month stretch in a particularly toxic work environment, I recall that I would instantly break out in hives every time my boss entered the room. I had never experienced this before. Since I was in such a high-alert state most of the time and I associated that person and place with feelings of resentment, anger, fear, and anxiety, my body responded according to the perceived threat (thanks to my amygdala). The hives were a warning sign that something was not right, and I needed to listen to the warnings in my body. Whether the figurative chicken or egg came first (a created association with this individual, or if my body was screaming that something was not safe for me), I was developing anticipatory stress responses in my body just at the mere presence of this individual.

To identify what triggers stress for you, be specific here - the who, what, when, where, and why. The extent of your stress association may surprise you. Ask yourself and write:

- **Who** are you with when you feel the most intense effects of stress? Is there a particular person who you respond to with stress in your body more often?

- **What** specific thoughts, events, beliefs, or emotions precipitate feelings of stress in the body?

These answers will differ for every person. For me, I feel more stress in my body when it feels like I have too much on my plate and not enough time to get it all done. Now, I rephrase this stressor is by saying, "I have the same 24 hours as every other human. I am going to pace myself so I can be efficient and not cause myself undue stress. The world will not end because I don't get the laundry folded today."

- **When** do you feel stress in your body? Is it every morning as you are getting ready to go to the job you despise? Is it every evening before you get home, anticipating the chores and arguments that you might have? Are the effects of stress more pronounced when you have not slept well, or when you have missed a meal or two?

For me, stress, and the ripple effect of that stress (lingering anxiety, lack of sleep, missing meals, etc.) caused 95% of migraines. I will share how I eliminated this response in my body in coming chapters.

- **Where** are you when you feel the most stress? At home, work, school, or with a particular group of people?

- **How** can you redirect the physical effects of a stressor in your body? When stress overcomes you, what can you control?

Sometimes it helps to respond to physical symptoms with counterpart physical actions, like regulated breathing. We can feel an emotion in our body, and we can have the conversation right back to our body and say, "Although I feel a tightness in my chest because I am uncertain about the outcome, it is not in my control - therefore, what I can control is the rate and depth of my breath."

- What is your internal dialogue that you are communicating to your cells throughout the day? If you spoke to a friend the way you speak to yourself, would your friend feel uplifted and motivated, or would they feel like giving up?

- Now imagine your friend represents the millions of cells in your body, working endlessly to keep you alive and well. What messages are your cells communicating back to you in the form of physical responses?

Our cells are listening to our thoughts - I really cannot emphasize that enough. What we say manifests itself in a language of vibration on the cellular level. If we say to ourselves, "I will never get better. I can never enjoy my life. I am an idiot. I will always have migraines. It's never going to get any better..." our bodies will not stand a chance. Now, while this self-talk is not the primary reason someone may experience disease or disorder, it is part of the cumulative effect of how we are communicating with the body we occupy. Proverbs 14:30 reads, "A sound mind makes for a robust body, but runaway emotions corrode the bones." A negative mindset is like a flat tire. You can't go anywhere until you change it.

>> Be mindful of the possessive phrases you use.

The number one sentence I challenge you to rephrase is "I have a migraine." If we cumulatively had a quarter for each time we said this phrase, we could all purchase our own island and retire comfortably. It was not until two years ago that I stopped saying "I *have* a migraine." I realized that the word "have" is possessive, and according to Webster, means to "possess, own, or hold." No, thank you! I chose to no longer "possess, own, or hold on to" migraines anymore. I changed the way I spoke about them, and I would encourage you to do the same. From this moment forward, instead of saying "I have a migraine," I challenge you to say out loud, "I am experiencing the symptoms of a migraine, such as pain in my eye and nausea. I am in control of my breathing. Although I feel these sensations in my physical body, I am not possessing or holding on to this migraine. It does not define me; I am experiencing the effects of changes in my body, but I am safe."

- Write the alternative way you will talk about migraines here. You could say an analogy such as, "When I stand in the rain, I can feel the rain, and it might even get my skin wet. But I am not the rain, and the storm will pass. I can choose how I respond to what I am experiencing."

The next time a negative thought comes into your mind, immediately reverse it. Take a stand for what you want to declare about your health. You have power to change the way you think about yourself. When you have a moment, look up the IKEA Plant Experiment. Spoiler alert: the plants that were spoken to positively for 30 days had a different outcome than the plants that were spoken to negatively.

Let's start here:

- Write a common phrase you say to or about yourself.

- Now, remove the "negative" and flip it to a positive, with a solution.

Example of a negatively focused statement:

"I will never enjoy the concert because I have a migraine."

Now, an example of a flipped statement:

"Although I am experiencing a migraine, I will do my best to enjoy the day I have been given and be present in my body during the concert. If I choose not to go to the concert, that is my choice, I am in control of how I spend my time."

I know it sounds rudimentary and cliche, there is power in words to rewire the brain- when done consistently. Positive thinking can be the default response. *Neurons that fire together, wire together.*

>> Identify your default stress reaction and replace it.

When pressures of life become too great for us to carry, we all have a default response to protect us from the stressor. There are a split two seconds between hearing bad news and then the warm tingling sensation in the chest where we can either continue, or consciously change.

I am going to be vulnerable for a moment. As a child, when I was scared or sad, I would run away and hide.. I remember hiding behind the couch at age seven when I heard people arguing. I ran away from home for two weeks at age 14. There have been occasions where I have packed my suitcase and thrown it in the trunk of my car after relationship stress became too heavy for me to bear. My default stress response has always been to run away or hide.

> *"Between stimulus and response there is a space.*
> *In that space is our power to choose our response.*
> *In our response lies our growth and freedom."*
> -Viktor Frankl

We are predominantly either **introspective** or **extrospective** stress responders. We either internalize our fears, anxieties, anger, or stressors, or we externalize them. I tend to internalize my stress response and retreat. Some people may reach for a glass of wine when they feel stressed (drinking wine is not the problem, it is under what circumstances we drink). Others may get angry and yell, throw things, or stomp their feet. Some people may cry and hyperventilate or reach for the cookie jar to help soothe the pain. What is your default stress response? It is important to identify it and ask yourself; is this response helping me, or is it hurting me?

Although running and hiding has not directly hurt me, it has hurt my relationships and my ability to face uncomfortable or painful situations. Part of conquering the migraine experience is doing the deep soul work of **introspection** (observation of emotional and mental processes and states) and **interoception**, which is sensing the internal state of the body. I will share more on interoception in the chapter *Yoga, Meditation, and Breath.*

- Write your default stress reaction.

- How does this reaction affect other areas of your life, such as your relationships, your job, your sleep, eating habits, finances, and the occurrence of migraines?

- Write an ideal stress response that you would like to adopt.

For me, this was communicating to my family the pressure of stress I felt, saying, "I am going to go into the bedroom and practice yoga for 15 minutes so I can calm down." This is a healthier alternative to running away or hiding. I am choosing the space, choosing a healthy activity, choosing a time frame, and communicating it externally (since I tend to internalize stress).

The next time you are feeling sensations of a migraine or changes in the areas of your body related to stress, try this new response immediately. *This takes practice and consistency!* Rewrite your self-talk script. Be present in your body and recognize your thought patterns. Observe how you feel emotionally or what your thoughts are right before the migraine symptoms started. Ask yourself, what part did I play in this migraine? You may experience a migraine, but you do not have to possess and hold to it. I know this part may be difficult - it was for me. My default response was always, "Why is this happening to me...? I hate this." However, it is your physiology at play, and it is important to shift your thinking to optimize balance in your mind-body. Changing our internal script takes time, consistency, and practice. Remember, you are in control of your response, even if it doesn't feel like it at first.

- Write down how migraines have made you feel, and how you will change the way you talk about the migraine experience to yourself or others here.

Chapter Six

Nutrition and Gut Health

Nutrition is more than what we eat, it is what we allow in our life.
-Elizabeth Priller

NUTRITION HAS BEEN SOMEWHAT OF A BUZZ WORD in the 21st century, with new 'miracle' diets being flung at every ailment, disease, and defect. Migraineurs are no exception, having experimented with everything from Paleo to keto to intermittent fasting, all with varying degrees of success - yet we still do not have a definitive answer for which way of eating offers the best results. I understand that a chapter on can-eats and can't-eats may be the last thing you want to read. It can be overwhelming to hear someone revamp your entire eating regime. With this in mind, there are a couple of things I want you to remember.

First, know that no matter what guidance I share here, you are still in control of what you allow in your life and your body. This is *your* wellness journey. You are the driver. Second, remember that what you choose to put on the end of your fork really does influence the quality of your physical, emotional, and mental health. That is why it is so important for me to include this chapter. I will challenge you to consider which areas of your life are lacking nourishment, not just the body but also your emotional, relational, or spiritual parts, as these can either promote or demote a proper balance in the mind and body. I believe nutrition is more than what we eat; *it is what we allow in our life*. Coupled with other lifestyle practices included in this book, nutrition plays a vital role in strengthening our physiological margin of resilience to stress, disease, and disorder.

During the first 27 years of my life, I went through perennial stages of eating fast food, heavy carbohydrate foods, high-sugar foods, coffee, and energy drinks. From age 14 and through age 27, I was diagnosed with Intractable and Hemiplegic Migraines, Celiac Disease, Irritable Bowel Syndrome, Lupus, Mixed Connective Tissue Disease, Anxiety, and Depression. Stress, trauma, and high functioning overcommitment were an everyday part of my life. I allowed toxic relationships in my life by failing to say "no" when situations or people did not feel right. I ate whatever was put in front of me that was fast and convenient. Now that I understand how these choices can manifest in the physical body, I believe that many of these diseases and disorders were warning signs of a potentially lethal path.

My precarious nutritional lifestyle came to a screeching halt in 2005 after I went swimming in a lake in Wisconsin. Of my family members who were also swimming in the lake, I was the sole lucky recipient of an intestinal parasitic infection, giardiasis. I was hospitalized a few days later with intractable diarrhea, vomiting, mild kidney failure, and elevated liver enzymes. After losing 15 pounds in one week, I was forced to reevaluate the toxic way I had been living; my choices were having on my health, and the way I felt in my body and mind. The parasite infection was not the cause of my health issues leading up to that period, but it forced me to take a serious inventory of what I was allowing in my life.

"Your blood work seems normal. I am not sure what is wrong."

Prior to the parasite infection, I had been experiencing brain fog, severe joint pain, incessant headaches and migraines, unintentional weight loss, undigested food in my bowel movements, extreme bloating to the extent that I appeared 5-6 months pregnant, abdominal pain akin to eating broken glass, alarming rates of hair loss, and sensations of tunnel vision and distorted hearing after eating certain foods. I had to put a heating pad on my abdomen after eating to relieve post-meal cramps. I realized this had become my new normal when every doctor I visited simply said, "Your blood work seems normal. I am not sure what is wrong." Over a trial-and-error period of about two years, I could discern what foods made me feel like last week's rotting garbage, and what foods seemed to pass through my gut without major repercussions. It was a long process, but one that was absolutely essential to my wellbeing moving forward. In this chapter's method, I will share with you ways to revitalize the gut, balance the microbiome, and optimize the gut lining, all of which will help reduce risk factors for migraine development.

Obesity and Migraines

What will become increasingly clear as you progress through this book is that lifestyle choices directly impact a person's likelihood of developing disease or disorder, such as migraines. As we have learned, the body constantly ebbs and flows to maintain balance. The liver stores glucose for when we skip a meal, and it releases a temporary dose into the bloodstream if we don't eat in time. When we overeat, the pancreas secretes a massive amount of insulin to bring our blood sugars down to baseline. Over time, these systems become overused, exhausted, and can cause disease or disorder (such as diabetes, obesity, heart disease). Dysregulated energy balances can also result in obesity because of increased consumption of energy and reduced energy expenditure. So why talk about energy balance, appetite, and obesity in a book addressing migraines?

Obesity poses a great risk for chronic migraines; while the state of being obese may not directly cause migraines, the lifestyle which accompanies it certainly can. Research shows an increased frequency and severity of migraines in people who have an increased body mass index (BMI) over 30, compared to people that are overweight (a BMI of 25-30) or of natural weight (a BMI of 18.5-25). Alarmingly, the percentage of obese Americans went from 30.5% in 1999 up to 42.4% in 2018. The largest age group of obese Americans consists of adults between 40-59 years old, followed by ages 60 plus, and then adults that are 20-39 years old. All three age groups have at least 40% that are considered obese, defined by a BMI greater than 30 (Hales, Carroll, Fryar, & Ogden, 2020). What this infers is that there are millions of Americans living the lifestyle conducive to gaining excessive weight - overeating, sedentary movement, and chronic stress. These are all behaviors which exhaust and harm the body and mind, increasing the risk of migraine development.

Stress, Cravings, and Appetite

To echo the previous chapter, *Stress and Emotions*, how we emotionally respond to the world around us - particularly chronic stress - affects our appetite and cravings. Perhaps you have experienced heartbreak, where it feels as though nothing will soothe the pain better than a bowl (or two) of ice cream. When stress hits at work or home, you may crave hot, salty, and starchy French fries. Why do we crave these types of foods? Stay with me, friend, as I unravel for you why we crave certain foods, especially when we are under stress.

As the effects of chronic stress invade our lives and the pressure mounts, we know that this results in an increase of the stress hormone cortisol. To complicate the layers of stress, increased cortisol also dramatically increases one of the hormones that controls appetite - **ghrelin**. This circulating "hunger hormone" makes us crave foods high in fat, carbohydrates, or sugar, and increases the risk for overeating. Ghrelin is also partially responsible for the appetite changes which occur before or after a migraine, which is why you may begin to crave carbohydrates at these times. Ghrelin is secreted in the stomach and sends signals from the gut to the hypothalamus in the brain, saying, "Feed me now!" This hormone also influences the sleep-wake cycle (circadian rhythm).

Here's a tip: when we are sleep deprived, ghrelin levels skyrocket. Think about what you crave when you are sleep-deprived - is it high fat, high carbohydrate, or high in salt? To balance ghrelin levels, avoid extremes in dieting and changes in weight, such as with Yo-Yo dieting or calorie restrictive diets. Some treatments for obesity focus all the attention on the food, when the best way to deal with ghrelin is to go straight to the root: improve your quality of sleep and create interventions to help manage stress. Increasing muscle mass through regular exercise will also help decrease out-of-control ghrelin levels.

Remember the vagus nerve? Well, we know it has receptors in the gut that communicate with the brain. Ghrelin communicates via the vagus nerve to the brain to *suppress* the sympathetic nervous system release of epinephrine and norepinephrine (stress, fight, or flight system). This may illustrate why we may feel calmer or more soothed after a high calorie, fat, salty, sugary, or carbohydrate meal. Increased release of the inflammatory molecules such as TNF-*a* and cytokines follow in the presence of ghrelin (unnecessary inflammation = one pillar of migraine occurrence).

The fraternal yet opposing twin of ghrelin that *decreases* the appetite is **leptin**. One way to remember how each one affects the appetite is G = Grow, L = Low. Leptin works as a "fat controller" by suppressing the appetite. Leptin threshold levels are genetically preset, and every person has a different "normal." Release of this appetite-suppressing hormone from fat cells in the body signals the hypothalamus to alter the amount of food intake. Leptin tells your brain you have enough energy in your fat cells to engage in sustained activity. When a person starves or severely reduces their calorie intake and loses body fat, leptin levels also drop. As a result, it turns the vagus nerve on to stimulate the appetite. Can there be too much of a good thing? Incidentally, the more body fat a person has, the more leptin that is circulating in the blood. It sounds as if this would suppress the appetite, but the brain becomes resistant to leptin and does not respond appropriately, signaling to eat more. This means that more body fat essentially leads to a larger appetite. We all have a bottom level threshold of leptin, but there is no ceiling threshold. What happens in obesity is the body has plenty of circulating leptin (because of increased fat cells), but the brain cannot see it and perceives the body is starving.

Footnote: Additional appetite hormones, Orexin A and B, are also involved with appetite and sleep/wake cycles. Production of these hormones occurs as a response to increased cravings for food and is associated with the condition narcolepsy.

Pulling Roots

Hippocrates, recognized as the Father of Medicine, was ahead of his time thousands of years ago when he practiced medicine under this principle: "Let food be thy medicine, and medicine be thy food." This quote gives control back to the person who is holding their fork and shines a light on the power of nutrition in the body. As a classically trained nurse in Western allopathic medicine, I was taught to seek treatment for symptoms, rather than finding and remedying the root cause of said symptoms. There is a critical flaw to solely using this practice: if I were to take an over-the-counter pain reliever, migraine abortive, or narcotic for every migraine I felt, without doing my due diligence in seeking to understand *my role* in the migraine's cause, I would only be treating the temporary pain associated with my chronic condition. In homeopathic or integrative medicine, on the other hand, we are taught to look at root origins, investigate non-drug therapies, and consider the *whole person* when managing symptoms; and nutrition is one of the most critical elements to consider. These two systems have a synergistic effect.

Envision that I am trying to remove a noxious weed from my garden. If I continue to only pull the leaves off the weed, the weed will continue to grow. However, I become an active participant if I take the investigative path and examine the roots, the soil, the conditions of the garden, and my negligence of consistently weeding the garden. I discover not only what the weed is, but why it is there, and how I can work to reduce its pervasiveness in my garden. Subsequently, I pull the weed out by the root so that it cannot grow deeper into the soil. This is the vital difference between the two medical practices; we can either pull at leaves and alleviate symptoms, or we can dig down to the roots and treat the underlying origins for a more sustainable effect. Sometimes, both are necessary to reduce suffering.

An integral part of digging the roots and investigating underlying causes is carried out by first inspecting the *gut*. In fact, gut health can be improved to reduce migraine occurrence. It is important to note that migraines are often associated with disorders of the gut such as Irritable Bowel Syndrome (IBS), Inflammatory Bowel Disease (IBD), Celiac Disease (CD), and a bacterial infection of the stomach that causes stomach ulcers,

H. Pylori. A randomized study showed that 45% of migraineurs participating in the study had the stomach bacteria *H. Pylori*, whereas it was found that only 33% of participants without migraines had an *H. Pylori* infection. Connections are shown between *H. Pylori* infection and increased levels of cytokines such as IL-10 and CGRP, which both aggravate the onset and severity of a migraine. *H. Pylori* also predisposes a person to be in a chronic, low-level inflammatory state, which we know can catalyze unrelenting chronic migraines. In addition, research shows that chronic migraineurs have a higher chance of being diagnosed with IBS than people without migraines.

The Microbiome, Gut Brain Axis, and Inflammation

The connection between the gut and the brain is through a bio-communication system called the **Gut-Brain Axis**. Messengers that communicate information reciprocally from the gut to the brain are inflammatory markers such as: TNF-*a* and IL-6, serotonin, CGRP, VIP, Neuropeptide Y, stress hormones, vitamins, and the individual's distinct microbiome. The **microbiome** is the genetic makeup, or **deoxyribonucleic acid (DNA)** of bacteria, viruses, yeast, and fungi that live in the gut, and are unique to each person. This communication occurs via the terminal ends of the vagus nerve that go from the brain to the gut, sending information both ways. As we balance the microbiome (the plethora of microbes that live inside of us), we are better able to build resilience of the vagus nerve.

The gut contains approximately ten times more microbes than all the cells in your body. DNA of the bacteria has information that guides our health, all the way from the gut to the brain. The microbiome and neurons in the gut are newly referred to as the "second brain", or the **enteric nervous system**.

The Microbiome and Leaky Gut

It makes for a healthy gut when there is a diverse pool of bacteria that work together for the benefit of all body systems. DNA is packed tightly in every cell, both bacteria and person. In the human cell, DNA is the messenger of genetic material that tells each part of the body what to do. Wrapped compactly in the cell is the genetic material that can be turned on based on environmental conditions, chemical exposures, stress, and - in the case of our gut - bacteria and what we eat. We refer to imbalances in gut bacteria as **dysbiosis**, where there is less "good" bacteria and more "bad" bacteria. Dysbiosis can occur due to chronic stress, prescription medications (such as antibiotics), over-the-counter drugs (such as ibuprofen, aspirin, and acetaminophen), excessive alcohol consumption, lack of food diversity, lack of physical activity, cigarette smoking, poor sleep, and low-level inflammation from chronic diseases. A fork crammed with inflammatory foods such as processed meats, dairy products, fried foods, and foods high in sugar also contribute to imbalances in the gut microbiome.

Dysbiosis and the accompanying lifestyle factors can degrade the functional lining of the gut and result in a condition called **leaky gut**

syndrome. Leaky gut syndrome is a group of symptoms that develop because of impaired gut permeability. The lining of the gut, primarily the small intestine, allows good things in and keeps bad things out (such as toxins, metabolic byproducts, and chemicals). Think of a healthy gut lining like a tightly woven fabric; it allows small micronutrients and water in, but keeps out large toxins, bacteria, and byproducts. With leaky gut syndrome, this tightly woven fabric develops larger openings, becomes inflamed, and ends up more loosely woven. The molecules that are not meant to enter the bloodstream now have access to the body, by way of the permeable gut lining, where they can cause further disruption, inflammation, and eventually, disease or disorder. The translocation of gut bacteria and inflammatory molecules entering the bloodstream can lead to systemic inflammation and the release of inflammatory cytokines, often leading to an activation of autoimmune conditions. Scientists have speculated for decades that a disrupted gut microbiome can contribute to the development of colon cancer.

Leaky gut may also result in a trigger of the trigeminal nerve pathway and the release of vasoactive peptide (VIP), which is the sister hormone to CGRP, activating a migraine. Symptoms of leaky gut syndrome include fatigue, headaches, chronic diarrhea or constipation, excessive bloating, food sensitivities, excess gas, confusion or brain fog, trouble focusing, joint pain, and skin problems such as psoriasis, rosacea, acne, rashes, hives, or other inflammatory skin conditions. We theorize that leaky gut plays a significant role in the development of autoimmune conditions such as Lupus, Crohn's disease, Rheumatoid Arthritis, Psoriasis, Multiple Sclerosis, and Hashimoto's Thyroiditis.

The Microbiome and Migraines

So how are the microbiome and gut health related to migraines? We know that the gut bacteria have DNA, and these DNA communicate to the brain about the status of the body. If there is an imbalance of beneficial vs. harmful gut bacteria (because of the causes previously mentioned), there may be disruptions in the information sent to the brain. Dysbiosis and leaky gut affect hormone production, mood, inflammation, sleep, and the body's ability to rid itself of toxins. CGRP, one of the primary inflammatory molecules involved with migraine induction, has been shown to alter the balance of gut bacteria. Inversely, imbalances in gut bacteria can influence activation of CGRP. An inequity of gut bacteria can also lead to activation of the HPA axis (homeostasis and hormone system) via the inflammatory molecules present in the gut. Low level chronic inflammation present in the body because of chronic stress, poor nutrition, lack of sleep, and a disrupted gut microbiome can set the stage for chronic migraines.

All of this is to say that impaired gut health is unswervingly associated with migraines. Our gut microbiome is so meticulously convoluted to our bodily functions; it only makes sense that an imbalance would set the stage for migraines, among many other health issues.

The Mind, the Brain, and Immunity

As we have learned, the systems of the body have symbiotic relationships. The gut, the brain, and the immune system all crave balance for our survival. Like the electrical wiring of a house, one blown fuse will affect everything beyond that fuse. One crooked wall will affect the functional structure of the entire house.

The body is in constant search for stability and will set off the alarm when it senses imbalance.

The branch of study that demonstrates this connection in the body is known as **psychoneuroimmunology**. Rest assured, the term is simpler than it looks; it is essentially the study of how the state of the mind affects our health and resistance to disease. The communication process between thoughts, emotions, gut health, and immunity is bidirectional, communicating up and down via the parasympathetic nervous system (rest and digest, via the vagus nerve) and the sympathetic nervous system (stress system).

In the previous chapter, we discovered how uncontrolled emotions can manifest as pain, fatigue, migraines, digestive issues, or other symptoms in the physical body. Tied closely to emotions is gut and immune health. You have likely heard the phrases, "trust your gut" or "gut instinct". These phrases have a grounding in science. Scientists have now determined that the gut-brain connection is deeper than a pie-in-the-sky hypothesis. We can describe a gut instinct as a physical feeling accompanied by a certain thought or emotion. Studies show that directly tied to gut health is the production of neurotransmitters such as **serotonin** (the happy hormone), **dopamine** (the pleasure hormone), and **gamma-amino-butyric acid** (GABA, a calming neurotransmitter). In fact, gut bacteria manufacture up to 90-95% of the body's serotonin - far more than the brain does. It is by no coincidence that many conventional migraine treatments, such as triptans and tricyclic antidepressants, focus on balancing serotonin levels. Nonetheless, the power lies in our ability to balance our gut bacteria and create a healthy environment to manufacture our own serotonin. A healthy gut encourages serotonin hormone production, which can then balance and optimize our moods, appetite, memory, sleep, and reduce the incidence of migraines.

The gut is the root of our immune system. By its insane bacterial manufacture rates, it renders us one-part human to ten-parts bacteria. Immune cells in the gut lining release antibodies into the gut, effectively promoting health and enabling us to fight off infection. Immune cells in the gut also have serotonin receptors which sit ready to accept or release serotonin. This is one demonstration of the mind-gut connectedness, and how it expresses the efficacy of the immune system through our mood.

Have you ever noticed that when you are not sleeping well, you tend to come down with a cold? Or, when you have an illness such as a cold, it lasts longer if you are not sleeping well? Perhaps you notice that prior to or during migraine, your mood shifts? Recall what is happening during sleep - the brain is restoring cells, hormones, and tissues. The gut works the same way. A healthy, balanced gut microbiome with a robust gut lining helps keep the immune and neurological systems resilient and functioning optimally.

One that takes medicine and neglects diet, wastes the skill of the physician.
- Chinese Proverb

Inflammatory Foods and Ingredients

Throughout my journey with migraines, I have had to play Russian Roulette with trying to find what foods worsened or triggered migraines. I am sure you can relate; the arduous trial and error process, cutting out your comfort foods, reacting poorly to foods you thought were healthy. Keep in mind that every person's biology is different, and we all can respond differently to the same ingredient. For example: some migraineurs are instantly triggered by caffeine, while others find it alleviates their migraines. This section is aimed at making the elimination process a little simpler by breaking down some of the leading food and ingredient triggers for migraines. I will explain how these ingredients work in the body, so that you can better understand how it may work in your body. It will be up to you to decide how you use this information, and what you may discover as a contributing factor to your migraine experience.

Gluten

I remember trying to re-introduce food again after the intestinal parasite infection, giardiasis. The day they discharged me from the hospital, my body was ravenous; I stopped at a local fast-food restaurant and ordered a burger with cheese. I will spare you the graphic details on what happened next, but what followed for days on end was a pattern of nausea after every meal. Any food I ate came right back up. The doctors and I both pinned this down to a recovering gastrointestinal system, figuring those heavier foods were just too much for my inflamed body to handle at the time. We were right in some respects; as it turned out, the parasite had ravaged my gut and left me with a temperamental immune system. It was now hyperreactive and acting like a two-year-old in a tantrum, rejecting all of the foods I was eating. The provisions I had been putting into my body for the previous 27 years no longer made the cut. In hindsight, this shift really was for the best - I needed a life-altering event to grab my attention and alert me of the ways I had been mistreating my body.

I was 27 years old when I first heard about gluten. Severely underweight at 103 pounds on a 5'6" frame, my body was not well. Over the next year of laborious trial and error, I was finally diagnosed with Celiac Disease amid multiple visits to the doctor. This diagnosis had an extreme impact on my life moving forward, completely changing my lifestyle and my perception of health.

Celiac Disease is an immune condition of the gut that occurs in the presence of wheat, gluten, and gluten-derivatives. We can think of **gluten**

as the "glue" protein that holds grains together, such as the stretchy binder of wheat, barley, oats, and in everyday foods like bread, pizza, pasta, cakes, pastries, crackers, salad dressings, and cookies. It is estimated that 1-3% of the population has true Celiac Disease, and upwards of two million people have undiagnosed Celiac Disease in the United States alone. When people with Celiac Disease ingest gluten, an inflammatory course develops, leaving behind a path of destruction in the small intestine. The damaged small intestine then leaves the person at risk of developing leaky gut. An abundance of inflammatory molecules and byproducts of food are then free to invade the body, while nutrients are not properly absorbed. Gluten intolerance is another form of gluten rejection in which the person may not have a severe immune response or allergic reaction, but instead does not properly digest gluten, and therefore cannot tolerate gluten in the diet. If a person with either of these conditions ingests gluten, the body reacts by fighting against the gluten protein with inflammation. The symptoms range from fatigue, brain fog, abdominal pain and bloating, constipation, diarrhea, or even migraines. For those that are diagnosed with Celiac Disease past the age of 20 (having consumed gluten for at least 20 years), there is a 34% increased chance of developing another autoimmune condition.

In the first month of being diagnosed with Celiac Disease, I thought that eating gluten was dose-dependent, meaning I could have a little and still be ok. I would eat Oreo cookies before bed and then hurriedly go to sleep as to not experience the inevitable symptoms. Low and behold, I would wake up an hour later with wringing abdominal pain, nausea, and occasionally vomiting. After eating my last gluten-tainted meal that left me feeling miserable, I finally made peace with my body rejecting gluten and eliminated the obvious sources of gluten from my diet. In only a few weeks I noticed a significant improvement of joint pain, hair loss, skin rashes, brain fog, abdominal pain, diarrhea, bloating, and migraines. The change was phenomenal. Before then, I had been experiencing at least 15-20 migraine days per month on average. In the first few months of eliminating gluten from my diet, I went down to about 5-10 migraine days per month. Going gluten-free did not eliminate migraine occurrence entirely, as I still had more work to do about what I allowed in my life. However, by alleviating underlying inflammation present in my body and beginning the gut healing process, there was a noticeable impact on the frequency of migraine attacks.

The effect that gluten had on my health became increasingly obvious to me as I paid more attention to the ways my body responded. Every time I would accidentally eat gluten, I noticed the other autoimmune conditions would "flare up." Rosacea and psoriasis would return, migraines would return, and the joint pain and fatigue from connective tissue disease would return. It would take 7-14 days for me to recover from ingesting an accidental crumb of bread or eating foods that had hidden sources of gluten. It became clear to me that even a small digression simply wasn't worth the aftermath. Taking control of my nutrition, I spent the next three years scrupulously reading food and drink labels, committing to memory the hidden sources of gluten and gluten-similar ingredients such as modified food starch, corn, oats, barley, and caramel color.

Research has shown that in patients with IBS, gluten intolerance, or Celiac Disease, food elimination diets may reduce the associated symptoms and reduce the occurrence of migraines. Some studies suggest that eliminating gluten from the diet may be effective in decreasing migraine frequency. So besides eliminating gluten, how can you restore gut health and the microbiome? Let's jump right into the next method.

Method #3: Regenerate the Gut and Reduce Inflammation

The nutritional lifestyles outlined in this step may help to improve migraine occurrence and severity, according to selected research and numerous testimonials. When approaching a nutritional plan that works best for your body, it is important to remember that everyone is different. We are unlikely to come across one wonder plan or magic diet that works for all migraine sufferers. Instead, we each must undertake our own personal investigation, using trial and error to eliminate the foods which exacerbate the migraine experience. In saying that, there is research to back the concept that some foods are inflammatory and will disrupt proper functioning of the gut. For example, foods that are highly processed will often pose an increased inflammation risk. When seeking the best nutrition for your body, one rule of thumb I find helpful is to try to consume food in its purest form wherever possible.

>> Gluten-Conscious or Gluten-Free Nutrition

If you choose to omit gluten from your nutrition, here are the names of potential gluten sources to look out for. Some of these foods may induce a similar reaction to gluten in the body.

Potential gluten sources:

Barley

Brewer's Yeast

Caramel Color

Corn, corn syrup (some people can tolerate corn and corn products)

Durum, Farrow, Semolina, Spelt, Farina

Gluten

Hydrolyzed Wheat Protein, Hydrolyzed Corn

Malt, Malt Vinegar

Matzo, Panko Breadcrumbs

Modified Food Starch

MSG (monosodium glutamate)

Oatmeal, oat bran, oat flour, whole oats (unless they are from pure, uncontaminated oats, some people can tolerate oats, some cannot)

Pregelatinized starch

Wheat, wheat germ, wheat flour, wheat starch

Yeast extract

Packaged Foods to Inspect and Avoid:

Processed foods or packaged foods

Sauces, dressings, marinades, gravy

Sausages, deli meats, processed meats

Soy sauce (unless gluten free)

Spices and seasonings

Beverages

Safe baking and flour alternatives:

Almond Flour

Arrowroot Flour

Buckwheat Flour

Chickpea Flour

Coconut Flour

Quinoa Flour

Sorghum, Teff, or Amaranth Flours

Xanthan Gum (baking "binder")

>> Plant-based, Vegan, Vegetarian, or Pescatarian

Meat is not bad; but more important is to uncover how the body processes meat. For example, red meat has substances that fresh fish or fowl do not have. The main culprit in red meat that may trigger a migraine is **tyramine**. Tyramine is an amino-acid that regulates blood pressure and heart rate, by signaling nerve cells to release adrenaline. Other foods that contain inflammatory compounds like tyramine are aged cheeses, most beers, cured or processed meats such as sausages, smoked fish, or caviar. In addition, a plant-based diet has been shown to reduce estrogen dominance, improve blood pressure control, and reduce cardiovascular disease risk. Dairy foods tend to be inflammatory in some people that have underlying chronic inflammation or food intolerances. It is known that **nitrate** compounds (used as flavor enhancers and preservatives) may cause migraines via a release of CGRP. Foods and beverages that contain nitrates such as wine, soy sauce, processed meats, pickled foods, and steak sauce contain nitrates and nitrites and may induce a migraine. Other substances such as **aspartame** and artificial sweeteners can increase levels of acidic amino acids in the brain and further irritate the nervous system.

Plant-based diets can range from a mostly plant diet to completely vegan (avoiding all animal-based products). Most importantly, make sure your diet is balanced, and full of rich and dark color fruits and vegetables such as greens, purples, blues, reds, oranges, and yellows. Naturally colorful foods are rich in antioxidants that help reduce oxidative stress in the body. Plant-based sources of protein include tofu, lentils, beans, and nuts. In a plant-based meal plan, 50% of the plate should be high quality vegetables such as broccoli, spinach, peppers, zucchini, beans, squash, pumpkin, or kale. Fresh herbs and spices such as turmeric, ginger, garlic, parsley, coriander, and curry can be beneficial and help reduce the risk of inflammation. Additionally, it is wise to avoid high glycemic foods that raise the blood sugar quickly, such as sugary baked goods, sugar-laden drinks, refined foods, sodas, and heavy carbohydrates such as pizza, breads, and pasta.

The four-letter F word that is imperative to the diet to balance health, regulate hormones, and decrease inflammation is *fats*. However, the type of fat is important to differentiate. The easiest way to remember what types of fats are superior for the body are fats that are liquid at room temperature, or plant based. These **unsaturated fats** include coconut oil (which contains some saturated fats), hemp oil, almond butter, olive oil, flaxseed oil, avocado oil, or sesame oil. Fats that are solid at room temperature tend to be animal-based and are considered **saturated fats**, which can increase inflammation and cardiovascular disease risk. These fats include butter, milk/cream, ice cream, lard, fat from meat, and egg yolks.

If you choose to adopt a plant-based or anti-inflammatory nutritional way of living and eating, give yourself three full months to observe for changes. Studies have shown that participants that followed a plant-based anti-inflammatory diet for three months had lower scores of migraine severity and frequency. Consistency will help you gauge how nutrition impacts migraines.

>> Balance the Microbiome

The first line of defense to boost the microbiome is to cut out toxic foods from your diet. Inflammatory foods such as the ones listed above can disrupt normal gut bacteria and permeate the gut lining. Reducing stress will also promote a balanced microbiome by reducing stress hormones and balancing appetite hormones. Increasing aerobic exercise can also promote a healthy gut microbiome. Sufficient high-quality sleep also promotes a healthy microbiome by reducing cravings and stabilizing mood neurotransmitters. Research shows that only two days of sleep deprivation can cause measurable changes to the gut microbiome and increase the load of bacterial strains associated with weight gain, obesity, and Type 2 Diabetes.

Digestive enzymes (individually known as protease, lipase, amylase, among others) can be taken in supplement form, and help to break down fats, carbohydrates, proteins, and fiber to ease the work of the gut. As you eat more healthy fats, these fats work with fiber-rich foods known as *prebiotics* to convert into **short-chain fatty acids (SCFAs)**, which feed the good bacteria in your gut. Prebiotics are foods such as garlic, shallots, spring onions, leeks, savoy cabbage, kimchi, kombucha, apple cider vinegar (with the "mother" strain), chickpeas, oats, lentils, kidney beans, bananas, watermelon, grapefruit, almonds, pistachios, flax seed, berries, chicory, and Jerusalem artichokes. These foods change the way and the rate your body breaks down food, especially sugars, which results in less blood sugar spikes. SCFAs also help protect the gut lining.

Probiotics are extra "good bacteria" that can help strengthen the gut permeability and reduce cortisol levels. Probiotics encourage the manufacture of short-chain fatty acids in the gut, which are beneficial for gut-brain homeostasis. Probiotics help diversify the gut microbiome, which can help augment the immune system. One study showed that when a strain of *Bifidobacterium Longum* bacteria was given to mice with pre-existing anxiety and intact vagus nerves, the bacteria stabilized their behavior to a calm state. These findings show how the vagus nerve acts as a gateway for the anxiety-reducing abilities of gut bacteria. Remarkably, some strains of probiotics support the conversion of tryptophan into serotonin (more on these neurotransmitters in the chapter, *Oxidative Stress and Dietary Supplements*). There are several strains of probiotics that have anti-inflammatory properties. This is important to recognize since CGRP levels have been shown to be higher in people with disrupted or imbalanced gut microbiomes.

Enhanced fitness levels have been associated with a greater proportion of **butyrate**, a short-chain fatty acid that's important for overall health. Research indicates that active women have a higher abundance of health-promoting bacteria, including *Bifidobacterium* and *Akkermansia*, suggesting that regular physical activity, even at low-to-moderate intensities, can be beneficial for gut health. (See Resources section for nutritional supplement brands.)

>> Low FODMAP

FODMAP, which is the acronym for "fermentable oligo-, di-, mono-saccharides and polyols" is a term describing the byproducts of certain carbohydrates that may produce inflammation and digestive issues such as bloating, gas, undigested foods, stomach pain, abdominal distention, and diarrhea or constipation. Some migraineurs find relief from avoiding these types of foods. *For more information on FODMAP diets, contact a dietician or your healthcare provider.*

>> Anti-Migraine Eating

Put simply, the best way to reduce migraine risk related to inflammation is to minimize or eliminate a) processed sugars, b) saturated fats, c) heavy carbohydrates, and d) processed foods. A good rule of thumb to eat *more from the earth and less from a box*. In addition to what you eat, though, it's important to focus on *how* you eat it. Do you find yourself watching television while eating dinner? Or scrolling social media feeds while eating breakfast? Worse yet, multitasking work while hurriedly eating lunch? Have you ever looked down at your plate after a meal and struggled to remember eating it, let alone enjoying it? These scenarios are examples of mindless eating, where our minds are busy in one direction, and our mouths are busy in another. Mindless eating can easily lead to overeating. Proper digestive functions are restricted when we are stressed, anxious, or angry. At one time, multitasking was praised, but now we recognize the significance of a mindful connection between our mood, mind, and meals.

A simple mindful eating exercise can be done during one meal of the day. Choose a meal that you tend to feel the most distracted, rushed, or disengaged. Prior to eating, take a deep breath and **check in** with your belly. How hungry are you on a 0-10 scale? Pause, and **evaluate** why you are choosing to eat right now. Next, **assess** your food using all your senses. What colors are in your food? How would you describe the textures of your food? Is the food hot, warm, or cool? What does it smell like?

After your first bite, **reassess** the food. How does it feel while you chew it? What other sensations do you notice in your body as you eat? Is the food as good as or worse than you expected? Next, **slow down**. So many times we are rushed, and our mealtimes tend to take on the same pace. **Set your fork down** in between bites and take ample time to chew your food thoroughly. This helps pre-digest your food and eases the work for the gut. Halfway through eating, take a moment to **investigate** your hunger level. Are you eating slowly enough for ghrelin and leptin to catch up to the brain? As you are eating, take time to **savor** your meal, fully experiencing the textures, colors, smells, and tastes. Allow these foods to **nourish** your body, and imagine each nutrient being broken down and delivered to your body right where it is needed.

Chapter Seven

Hormones and Neurotransmitters

A pure heart and mind only take you so far.
Eventually the hormones have their say, too.

- Jim Butcher

WHEN WE THINK OF HORMONES, what may come to mind are the familiar two sex hormones, estrogen and testosterone. The human body is entirely more complex than two yin and yang hormones, which are both present in a male and female. However, estrogen and testosterone play a major role in migraines across the lifespan of both sexes. If you are female, perhaps you have experienced a migraine at certain times throughout the month; occurring around ovulation or a few days before your menstrual period. This is just one example of the role hormones play in migraine occurrence. In this chapter, I will discuss how hormones and other biochemicals play a role in migraine development, what to do if these chemicals are out of whack in the body, and how to minimize hormone-related migraines.

Estrogen, Progesterone, and Testosterone

Migraines are more common in females, emerging at a 3:1 ratio compared to men. The peak occurrence of migraines in females is during the reproductive years (ages 18-29), with 43% of women experiencing migraines during this timeframe. Migraines in females frequently start with the onset of puberty and tend to wane after menopause. However, estrogen is not a female-only hormone. Men and women both have circulating levels of **estrogen** or **estradiol**, but estrogen levels in men are steadier throughout their lifespan. Women have fluctuating estrogen levels starting in puberty, monthly during the menstrual cycle, during pregnancy, in the postpartum period, with hormonal birth control use, and across the lifespan towards menopause, when estrogen levels plummet. In fact, a man of the same age as a menopausal woman has about three times as much estrogen. It is the more the zig zag variance of estrogen levels that precipitate a migraine, not just the overall falling levels of estrogen.

Symptoms associated with low estrogen include brain fog, memory changes, depression, insomnia, headaches (or migraines), dry vaginal tissue, weight gain, irregular periods, hot flashes, urinary leakage, or bone loss. Imbalanced estrogen can cause problems such as heavy menstrual bleeding, tender and sore breasts, severe premenstrual syndrome (PMS), cystic breast tissue, weight carried in the abdomen, anxiety or irritable moods, water retention and bloating, and increased triglyceride levels (high cholesterol). Lifestyle choices can affect hormone levels. In a female that does not consume enough healthy fats or calories, has extreme low body fat percentage, or undergoes extreme exercise, these can deplete her estrogen levels, which can then cause a missed or absent menstrual period. Fat cells account for about one-third of estrogen production in the body.

A sister hormone to estrogen is **progesterone**, which works with estrogen to help regulate the menstrual cycle and prepare the uterus for a fertilized egg. These two hormones fluctuate throughout the monthly cycle along with **luteinizing hormone (LH)** and **follicle-stimulating hormone (FSH)**, but it is the rollercoaster levels of estrogen that predisposes one to a hormone-related migraine. Females also have circulating **testosterone** produced in the ovaries at different levels than males. Testosterone's primary purpose in the female is to control the sex drive. As a woman nears menopause, testosterone levels drop, which can trigger a lower libido or sex drive. Too much testosterone production can interrupt a normal menstrual cycle, and can be related to high levels of insulin, also known as **insulin resistance**. This can occur for a myriad of reasons, but frequently diet, obesity, genetics, and other lifestyle habits play a significant role in the body's release of insulin. These imbalances may present themselves in the female body as excessive body hair, acne, and fertility issues such as in Polycystic Ovarian Syndrome (PCOS).

To help illustrate how these hormones work in a normal menstrual cycle, please see the table on the next page.

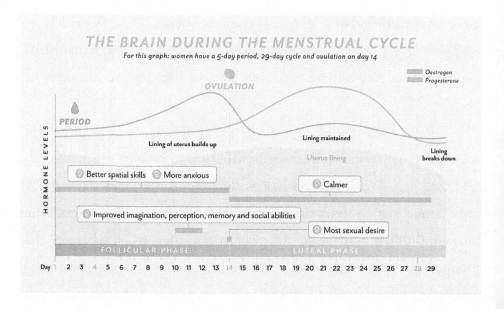

The Brain During the Menstrual Cycle, Image by Yoko Miyagawa/BBC, (Reprinted from Gorvett, 2018.)

We consider day one of the menstrual cycle as day one of the period. From the first day of the period to ovulation (around day 14), the ovary releases the egg in response to rising estrogen levels for potential fertilization. Estrogen levels peak around ovulation, then drop most severely right after ovulation, and again before the period. These hormonal shifts can cause symptoms related to PMS which can cause changes in the mood, bloating, breast tenderness, headaches, diarrhea, and changes in the skin. Reciprocally, progesterone rises, then drops right before the period from ovulation to the first day of the period. Testosterone slowly rises throughout the menstrual cycle, peaking during ovulation. The biological reason for this is to increase a woman's sex drive during her most fertile period to optimize the chance of a fertilized egg.

The Menstrual Cycle and Pain Sensitivity

During a woman's menstrual period, the uterus sheds the thickened lining when fertilization of the egg does not occur. During this time, **prostaglandins** are released from the lining of the uterus. Prostaglandins are chemical messengers that cause changes to the cells, such as initiating cramping to release the lining of the uterus (the period). However, the release of prostaglandins at the site of tissue "damage" (shedding of the uterine lining) can produce inflammation, pain, and occasionally a low-grade fever. Although this is a normal part of the tissue healing process, elevated prostaglandins also cause increased overall pain sensitivity, which can heighten the perception of pain during a menstrual period. In Chapter Nine, I will share the number one plant-based supplement that works to decrease the painful effects of prostaglandins and symptoms of PMS, which can support hormone balance and ease menstrual migraines.

Estrogen and the Brain

As we know, the brain is the central processor and the site for migraine development. So how do estrogen and genetic differences affect the migraine brain? For one, studies show that women with migraines have a thicker **insula** than male counterparts (and women without migraines). This research finding theorizes that being a woman migraineur predisposes her to changes in the brain structure and function, as well as neurological sensitivity. As a review, the insula processes basic survival sensory input such as taste, sensation, pain, pressure, sounds, light, and movement. The insula also regulates the sympathetic nervous system (automatic processes related to fight or flight) and the parasympathetic nervous system (automatic processes related to rest and digest), regulates and processes emotions, and plays a noteworthy role in activation of the immune system. Knowing what the insula controls and that this area is thicker in female migraineurs, suggests the connection between the extreme sensory and emotional changes experienced by women with migraines.

Moreover, estrogen also proliferates the production of **nitric oxide**, which is a potent vasodilator (widening) of cerebral arteries. We can equate low serotonin (which occurs at different times of the cycle) to more free roaming nitric oxide, which can correspondingly induce vasodilation and precipitate a migraine. On the other side, adequate serotonin levels actively lower CGRP and oppose excessive nitric oxide.

To tie it all together, let's go back to the trigeminal nerve, the largest and most complex of the cranial nerves associated with migraines. Research shows that there are estrogen receptors on the ends of trigeminal cells. Does this make it seem that women are automatically more predisposed to migraines via this channel, if the trigeminal nerve is ready to receive bits of estrogen? To no surprise, there are findings that link estrogen to the powerful vasodilator CGRP. In a study measuring hormone concentrations of rats, researchers found that low levels of estrogen tend to alter the concentration of CGRP (Aggarwal, Puri, & Puri, 2012).

Oxytocin

We often refer to **oxytocin** as the "love" or "bonding" hormone. The brain releases this hormone in the hypothalamus of both sexes, but its effects seem to be more dominant in a female. Oxytocin peaks during pregnancy, labor, breastfeeding, and triggers sexual orgasms. Researchers have linked higher levels of oxytocin to reduced migraine frequency. Similarly, some women report that sex provides migraine relief, and other female migraineurs report fewer migraine attacks while pregnant and during breastfeeding. For those that experience migraines during or after sexual activity, it could be due in part to vascular blood flow changes in the head, versus fluctuating oxytocin levels. In one case study of a pregnant woman experiencing a severe migraine, an infusion of oxytocin during labor induction anecdotally eased her migraine pain.

GABA

Oh, dear GABA, how do I love thee? Let me count the ways. **GABA,** also known as **gamma-amino-butyric acid,** is the principal inhibitory neurotransmitter that is biologically responsible for the state of calm. GABA inhibits stress hormones and neurotransmitters, which can reduce anxiety. This tranquilizing neurotransmitter also reduces overactivation of the HPA axis (center hub for stress monitoring, hormone release, and migraines). GABA promotes less stress reactivity, which means the same stressor produces less of a reaction in the presence of GABA. Many anti-anxiety medications such as lorazepam and clonazepam work on GABA receptor sites, but often with side effects such as grogginess, dry mouth, fatigue, constipation, and blurred vision. Incidentally, the practice of yoga increases GABA, and the effect can last for hours, helping maintain a blissful state of calm.

Serotonin

Estrogen is also partially responsible for changing levels of **serotonin** (the happy hormone) in the brain, which can alter pain sensitivity. In the presence of increased estrogen, serotonin levels are increased. However, when the lower levels of serotonin are present with decreased estrogen levels in the second half of the menstrual cycle, this blend can cause mood shifts towards depression, anxiety, poor outlook, and lethargy. These hormonal shifts predispose a woman to migraines during the second half of the menstrual cycle leading up to the period.

Low serotonin levels can turn on the migraine cascade.

Serotonin is also a powerful vasoconstrictor, which is narrowing of the arteries. As expected, drops in serotonin trigger vasodilation, which is a widening of the blood vessels. Think back to earlier chapters about the three chief causes of migraines- inflammation, vasodilation, and an overexcitable neuroelectric system. Low serotonin levels can initiate the migraine cascade by granting a widening of the blood vessels in the brain and body. Low serotonin levels also account for the accompanying anxiety, depression, or low mood during a migraine attack. *Yes, your mood and migraines are deeply connected.* To further illustrate the gut-brain-mood connection, many people experiencing a migraine often say that the migraine improves after vomiting. One reason for this mood change is that vomiting stimulates the gastrointestinal system to raise serotonin levels. Normal levels of serotonin support a brain free from the grip of migraines. Evidence also suggests that the depletion of the amino acid **tryptophan**, a precursor to serotonin, can exacerbate the symptoms of a migraine.

Tryptophan

Sometimes referred to as the "turkey hormone," **tryptophan** is a powerful amino acid that functions as a hormone and is more complex than its nickname. Tryptophan is an amino acid that is the "pre-hormone" necessary to manufacture serotonin. Tryptophan is found naturally in foods such as pumpkin seeds, chicken, eggs, peanuts, fish, milk, cheese, and turkey. I want to be clear- turkey does not directly raise serotonin levels. The process of tryptophan converting into serotonin is more complex. For this book, I will highlight these essential hormones to help build the framework of how they influence migraine development, or how they help avert migraine development. Bottom line, tryptophan is necessary to produce serotonin, which is essential to uplift our moods and mediate estrogen. Tryptophan also helps transcend a state of calm, which can reduce feelings of anxiety and promote quality sleep. Stay tuned for the chapter on dietary supplements where I impart how I have used tryptophan to consistently balance moods, promote healthy sleep, and keep migraines at bay.

Melatonin

Notorious for being known as the sleepy hormone, **melatonin** goes beyond just making us sleepy (referring to natural biological melatonin, not the over-the-counter supplement). Besides a preparatory signal for sleep, this powerful brain hormone acts as a free-radical scavenger. **Free radicals** are pernicious byproducts of chemical reactions in the body that, if left to circulate the body, can lead to inflammation, cell death, disease, and early aging. Melatonin helps mobilize antioxidant enzymes that scour free radicals. Think of melatonin as the cheerleader to the basketball team. As a bonus, melatonin blocks inflammatory signaling pathways, reducing inflammation particularly in the brain. There is more to come on melatonin in the next chapters.

As we learned in the chapter on sleep, melatonin is photosensitive, stimulated by light in the natural circadian rhythm. For example, in the brains of those ravaged by Alzheimer's disease, a protein called **beta-amyloid** is superabundant. Melatonin helps sweep up and destroy these sticky proteins in the brain, postulating that consistent quality sleep may ward off clumping of beta-amyloid. Not only does melatonin synchronize healthy sleep cycles, but it also supports the regulation of mood, immune system reactions, bone growth, hormones, and the suppression of tumors. This powerful anti-oxidant also is a key player in reducing inflammation and has neuroprotective effects (aiding in protection of the brain and nervous system via the immune system, after injury or inflammation). Melatonin is ten times more powerful than the antioxidant vitamin E and can help delay cellular aging. Some studies show that melatonin may support fighting bacterial, viral, and parasitic infections.

There are melatonin receptors widely distributed throughout the body, present in the heart, arteries, gut, endocrine (hormone) systems, reproductive system, and even in the skin. This shows that changes in melatonin levels can affect many systems simultaneously. And with what we know about the body's desire to be in a state of balance, when melatonin levels are low, the effects are experienced in multiple systems, including the brain.

Melatonin also blocks COX-2, which is an enzyme responsible for inflammation in the body. By blocking COX-2, melatonin helps decrease pain perception (i.e., migraines). At the cellular level, melatonin helps protect against dysfunction of the **mitochondria**, or energy powerhouse of the cell. (More to come on the vital role healthy mitochondria play in the management of inflammatory conditions, such as migraines, in the next few chapters.)

Now before you go out and buy a pallet of synthetic melatonin tablets, let's review the cycle of these hormones: tryptophan is the precursor to melatonin, and melatonin is the precursor to serotonin. Theoretically, if we have enough tryptophan to manufacture melatonin, we will have enough melatonin to produce serotonin. All three hormones work together to create a balance of mood, immune function, sleep, and quell inflammation, all of which are critical to the prevention of migraines. Perhaps you have tried melatonin in supplement form and found over time, it stops aiding your sleep. One hypothesis here is that, again if we look at root cause and support the predominant core hormone, other hormones are more likely to fall into balance.

Cortisol, Stress, and Hormones

Cortisol is synonymous with stress, but not all cortisol and all stressors are bad. In a well-balanced system, the natural release of cortisol by the adrenal glands happens at around 6 a.m. every day. To mirror what I shared in the chapter *Stress and Emotions*, the adrenals also release cortisol during periods of extreme or sudden stress to prepare the body for immediate fight or flight. In the immediate stress period, cortisol narrows the arteries, increases blood pressure, and floods the bloodstream with fat (triglycerides) and glucose. This sets the stage of how stress can create the perfect storm for a risk of neurological or cardiac events, such as a stroke or heart attack. Besides the obvious inflammatory storm of migraines, chronic stress without the execution of "fight or flight" eventually leads to insulin resistance, weight gain, inflammation, and chronic diseases. Soaring levels of the stress hormone cortisol over time increase the appetite for high carbohydrate and high-calorie foods by binding to receptors in the hypothalamus, fraudulently stimulating the appetite to correct imbalances caused by chronic stress.

Cortisol is an **immune system suppressant**, which initially is advantageous to keep an appropriate response to foreign invaders. Unfortunately, chronic stress can lead to a dysfunctional stress response, burned out adrenal glands, and an atypical immune response. Chronic inflammation stems from lifestyle habits such as inadequate diet, high levels of chronic stress, lack of consistent exercise, increased alcohol intake, smoking, and other daily behaviors that keep cortisol levels soaring dangerously. High cortisol levels can also increase the risk for cardiac diseases related to narrowing of the arteries and the buildup of plaque in the arterial walls. Over time, increased blood pressure, narrowing of the arteries, chronic inflammation, unhealthy lifestyle habits, and a disordered stress response will prove too much a person to stay well. Perpetually elevated cortisol levels can additionally lead to a higher risk of cancer, colds, opportunistic infections, food allergies, and autoimmune conditions such as Lupus, Rheumatoid Arthritis, Multiple Sclerosis, Psoriasis, Rosacea, Celiac Disease, Crohn's Disease, or Hashimoto's Thyroiditis.

Issues with fertility can arise from chronic stress related to a disruption in reproductive hormones. Since we produce sex hormones such as estrogen and progesterone in the same areas of the body as stress hormones, a surplus of cortisol can damper the production of normal sex hormones. Think about it, would anyone feel an inclination to have sex and procreate when a saber-toothed tiger is prowling nearby? The body knows no difference in threat.

Cortisol deactivates the parasympathetic nervous system (rest and digest) and activates the sympathetic nervous system (stress) which results in an impaired system. Only one division of the automatic nervous system can be dominant at any given time, so if the stress system is active, the rest system is dormant. Although these nervous systems are automatic, there are parts that *we can control*, such as our response to stress through regulating the breath. I will teach you effective breathing techniques to habitually activate the rest and digest system, which can reduce the severity and occurrence of migraines. We can promote balanced cortisol levels by managing our response to stress, prioritizing sleep, incorporating physical movement into our day, and eating an array of anti-inflammatory foods, all which help to recalibrate hormones.

Histamine

Remember, hormones and neurotransmitters in themselves are not harmful to the body, it is the balance of these chemicals that makes the difference in wellness versus illness. I would like to discuss a lesser-discussed neuromodulator, **histamine**, and its role in migraines. Histamine is a molecule that is released in response to a perceived or actual injury, allergy, or inflammation in the body. This may sound familiar from the class of medications called "antihistamines," such as the common medication Benadryl (diphenhydramine). You may start connecting the dots if you have ever had the migraine cocktail of Benadryl, Compazine (for nausea), and/or Toradol (for pain). Why does an antihistamine help ease migraines? Well, let's examine the role of histamine in the body, specifically with migraines. Again, if we know root cause and relationship to migraine development, perhaps we can avoid this imbalance.

Histamine modulates gut-brain axis activity and influences the release of other hormones that trigger migraines, such as CGRP and VIP. As with any other biological chemical, it can be over-secreted which leads to a neurological overreaction. In its best intent, when we are exposed to an allergen such as a bee sting, histamine is helpful to alert us of the threat. Recall, the body is in a constant state of protection and balance for survival.

Overproduction of histamine is common in migraineurs for several reasons. First, migraineurs can have a deficiency of the enzyme **diamine oxidase (DAO)**, which breaks down excessive histamine. In many circumstances, we can relate the overproduction of histamine or diminished DAO function to genetic variations, alcohol intake, medications, imbalanced gut bacteria, or the consumption of histamine-containing foods. Histamine is naturally present in several foods such as cheese, alcohol (beer, liquor, and wine), smoked or processed meats, fermented foods such as kimchi or kombucha, shellfish, dairy, wheat/gluten, peanuts and other tree nuts, strawberries, tomatoes (which also contain natural MSG), avocados, eggplant, spinach, and most preservatives, colors, dyes, and food additives. The first line to reduce migraine occurrence in those sensitive to the histamine response is by making dietary changes and not eating foods high in histamine.

While I did not highlight every hormone and neurotransmitter known to be present in the human body, the most common ones were brought to light. Hormones can be tricky to regulate as they are constantly changing. From our circadian rhythms to our biological age, hormones always have a say.

Method #4: Balance Your Hormones

As you work on balancing the other systems of the body through proper sleep and nutrition, your body will likely start to self-calibrate and restore normal hormone levels. If you have a coexisting disorder that affects hormone regulation such as PCOS or thyroid disease, you may find that these conditions convalesce as you stabilize your overall health. See your physician or other care provider for other specific hormone tests or balancing suggestions.

Chapter Eight
Genetics, Environment, and Lifestyle

Genetics play a huge part in who we are. But we also have free will.

-Aidan Quinn

WE ARE ALL BORN WITH A DISTINCT SET OF GENES that serve as the blueprint for our life. Consider these sets of genetic instructions as the owner's manual of our personality, physical characteristics, and ultimately, our health. The genetic blueprint is in the form of a deoxyribonucleic acid (more commonly known as DNA). Many times, I have heard people say, "I have high blood pressure because my father did," or "I am overweight because everyone in my family is overweight, it's in our genes." While the passing down of genes through families does indeed take place, we can influence our DNA expression through our choices. The foods we choose to eat, how much sleep we get, and what chemicals we expose ourselves to can turn our genes on or off. Our lifestyle choices activate DNA expression. This is such a freeing truth, as it means we have the power to change our quality of life.

Epigenetics

How often have you been likened, visually or otherwise, to one or both of your parents? When people say, "Wow, you look just like your father did when he was your age!" or "You sound exactly like your mother over the phone - I can hardly tell a difference!", they are observing traits that have been genetically passed down to you. Most of us carry this basic understanding of how genes are passed from parent to child. For example: I can observe that I have inherited my brown eyes, nose shape, and preference for spicy foods from my father, whereas my height, introverted personality, and small wrists likely came from my mother. These examples are the most foundational expressions of genetic material that we can see.

Epigenetics takes the study of gene expression and DNA a step further, building upon our basic knowledge of inherited genes. It explores other genetic features, like predispositions to certain health conditions, which can be silenced without affecting a person's actual DNA sequence. These are the genes which we can turn on or off to transform our quality of life. It can be tricky to understand this concept, so I will use a toggle switch metaphor to help simplify it.

Imagine you are in a room with a switchboard of 100 toggle switches. Each of these switches represents inherited genetic patterns of DNA from your biological mother and father. With our health, for example, we may have inherited from our parents a risk for heart disease, high blood pressure, cancer, diabetes, kidney disease, migraines, macular degeneration, or strokes. We categorize these examples as our family history; genes that are passed from generation to generation, increasing our personal risk for disease. Mentally picture those diseases and risks as switches on the control panel. Now, think about how the switches in a house operate; if I want light in the living room, I will turn on the switch for the living room. If I want to keep the kitchen dark, I will not turn on the switch for the kitchen. Our genes work in a very similar way - although we are born with genetic predispositions for certain diseases (the switches), some of us will see those diseases expressed in our bodies and some will not, depending on whether the genes are turned on or turned off.

For example, thanks to my father's genetic makeup, I have a risk for high blood pressure, but due to lifestyle choices, I consistently have a low blood pressure measurement of around 90/50. My grandmother died of Type 2 Diabetes complications, but I do not have diabetes, and instead have consistently have normal glucose levels. **Gene expression** can turn on just as a switch turns on a light. When the genes for various disorders and diseases are flipped on, we see the expression of the disease in the body. So, the question is this: what flips the switch?

How you choose to live your life can change your DNA.

DNA methylation is the efficiency of DNA and other cellular processes to complete necessary tasks such as hormone balance, detoxification, histamine clearance, cellular metabolism, gene expression, and immune cell activation. For most genes, more methylation is equal to a gene being turned "off" (also known as gene silencing), and less methylation is equal to a gene being turned "on." A person has better health equanimity and less disease risk if there is more methylation occurring. Several lifestyle factors alter the pattern of gene expression and can turn on or turn off genes (methylation) and expedite cellular aging. These lifestyle factors that rapidly increase disease risk include poor dietary choices, lack of physical activity, smoking, obesity, alcohol consumption, chronic psychological stress, working night shifts, and repeated exposure to chemicals or toxins. Indicators of low DNA methylation can be fatigue, mood changes, depression, anxiety, intolerance for histamine, increased development of cancer (because of genes being turned "on" for mutations and "off" for killing cancer cells), poor natural detox ability, infertility issues, and hormone imbalances.

Lifestyle Behaviors

If a person has the gene for colon cancer and they eat foods high in saturated fats, processed meats, preservatives, and drink alcohol, those lifestyle choices may "turn on" the gene for colon cancer to develop in their body. If that same person had the gene for colon cancer and ate a plant-based diet, consumed only low-inflammatory foods, avoided alcohol and tobacco, exercised regularly, and managed chronic stress, they may never develop colon cancer. With that being said, I recognize that there are various forms of disease with a myriad of causes, some of which we cannot change. However, I stand firm that if we allegorically inherit ten genes for disease, in theory we have the power to change eight of them through lifestyle choices. Why wouldn't I want to do my part in controlling my DNA expression?

Alcohol and tobacco are "co-carcinogens," which means they boost the harmful effects of cancer-causing agents. To illustrate, a person who has the gene for lung cancer who smokes tobacco will increase their risk of lung cancer, as the tobacco ingredients enhance mutations in lung cells. As aforementioned, lifestyle behaviors are some of the strongest influencers of DNA methylation. Researchers have observed drastic changes in DNA in people that smoke, drink alcohol, have poor nutrition, and have increased levels of chronic psychological stress.

Migraines and Epigenetics

While the causes of migraines vary for each person, there are genes directly involved with an increased risk of migraine development. Studies have shown that gene mutations for some migraineurs appear to speed up the excitability of the cerebral cortex (the brain structure involved in cortical spreading depression). This genetic predisposition to hyperexcitability is further expressed (turned on) in the presence of certain triggers such as stress, lack of sleep, inadequate nutrition or hydration, or hormone fluctuations. Genetic variations can also exist in vascular cells that control the dilation or contraction of blood vessels. Research shows there are nearly 20 irregular or mutated chromosome segments that are associated with migraines. To illustrate, if a person has the gene for a hyperexcitable cerebral cortex and then experiences a trigger such as a traumatic or stressful event that turns on that gene, this may be enough to turn on the gene for migraines.

Environment

Metaphorically, "we feed off of what is in our fish tank." One of the most primitive conditions that affects our DNA is our physical setting. Whether you read this book in your bed, at your desk, or at the local coffee shop, your location will directly influence how you feel and how your brain interprets your surroundings. Similarly, since our cells are listening and responding to every move we make, our physical location affects the way our DNA behaves.

Let's use the example of a mother's womb, since being in the womb for the first months of our development is a universally shared experience. The health habits, hormones, disease status, and nutrition of your birth mother all influence your development as a fetus in a sequence of events called **fetal programming**. Now, while this sounds like the brainchild of a computer scientist, fetal programming is the biological change that a fetus undergoes during development; the figurative switches are turned on and off, depending on how the development of the fetus is influenced. Studies show that during fetal development, a fetus' DNA blueprint is more susceptible to environmental changes due in part to its rapid growth in utero.

By changing our epigenetic signature, we may alter the genetic code that is passed down to our offspring.

After a baby is born, the environment he or she is born into further makes a difference in the expression of genes. DNA is constantly interpreting the environment and changing its activity based on cues from the environment. If a baby was born into an environment that is clean, orderly, calm, stable, and loving, that child's cells may not "turn on" the gene for a hyperactive fight-or-flight reaction, since it was likely not used much during the formative years. A child born to a drug-addicted mother in a home that is unstable, neglectful, chaotic, and in disarray may have to "turn on" the gene for fight-or-flight survival. Childhood trauma (indirectly witnessed or directly experienced) also influences how the child responds to stress later as an adult. These adverse childhood experiences (ACE) are associated frequently with migraines in adulthood, implying that childhood stress is linked to changes in the brain.

Childhood trauma and chronic stress can predispose changes in gene expression.

Early exposure to psychological stress can also predispose a person to overexpression of a gene receptor for stress hormones. In a study of suicide victims who had a history of experiencing child abuse, researchers found hyper-methylation (overexpression) of the gene for stress hormones, but this gene was *not found* in suicide victims who did not have a history of abuse in childhood. Another study revealed that the highest predicting link of migraines related to childhood abuse is specifically with emotional abuse. Those that reported childhood emotional abuse were 50% more likely to develop migraines in adolescence or adulthood. If a person experienced physical, sexual, and emotional abuse collectively, the risk of migraine doubled (Anda et al., 2010). Our experiences with stress and trauma affect the way we process stress, both physically and psychologically.

Environmental Toxins

Changes in DNA expression can occur in the presence of environmental toxins such as:

- heavy metals
- organic compounds (such as aromatic compounds, sulfates, and formaldehydes)
- pesticides
- air pollution
- endocrine (hormone) disrupters (such as chemicals found in plastics, antibacterial soaps, cosmetics, and detergents)

Chemicals can induce changes in the biochemical structure of DNA, leading to mutations in cells or alterations in gene expression. This means that people who frequently work with chemicals, such as gas station attendants, factory workers, hair or nail beauticians, construction workers, or painters may have a higher risk of cancer due to rapid cellular mutation, gene expression, and premature cellular aging.

Occupational environment such as shift work also penetrates gene expression. As we have learned about the connection between a natural circadian rhythm and quality of sleep, those that work night shifts may have changes expressed in their DNA that cause accelerated aging and inflammation. A study of night-shift workers showed they had impaired DNA methylation, specifically in the genes that turn on inflammatory markers such as TNF-*a*. From what we know about inflammatory markers and migraine development, this suggests that, besides disruptions in sleep, working the night shift can increase one's risk of chronic migraines due to inflammation at the cellular level.

90% of gene expression is related to lifestyle choices. 10% is related to heredity.

Individual Characteristics

The good news is that no two people are entirely biologically similar - not even identical twins. In fact, the Danish Twin Study, one of the most longstanding studies of health and longevity, summarizes that 80-90% of our health is related to **lifestyle choices** and **environment**, while 10-20% is related to **heredity**. Wow, had you ever considered that before? We have more control over our health than we may realize.

We all have biological, physical, emotional, and mental characteristics that separate us from being a carbon copy of another human. A 48-year-old black female who lives in a rural community and 22-year-old white male who lives in an urban area both have thousands of variants that separate how gene expression occurs. Our age, sex, geographical location, habits, personality type, and predetermined genetic blueprints determine how our cells respond to changes in our environment.

Do alterations in DNA end with *our body-mind*, or are we able to pass on to traits to our descendants for how they adapt to changes in the environment? Research shows that we can pass on to our children how to respond to the environment physically, emotionally, and mentally. One of the most fascinating studies of how DNA changes in response to the environment is a study conducted by scientists at Emory University, using mice and the smell of cherry blossoms. In this experiment, researchers used techniques of operant conditioning to teach male mice to associate mild electrical shocks with the smell of cherry blossom. They exposed the mice to the scent of cherry blossom for three days while experiencing the gentle shocks. Weeks later, the researchers bred the male mice with female mice that had not experienced the cherry blossom experiment. They found the most astonishing results in the offspring of these bred mice. The new offspring were born with neurons that detected the odor of cherry blossom, and when exposed to this odor, the offspring mice were jumpier, easily startled, and exhibited signs of fear (Dias and Ressler, 2014).

Epigenetics empowers you to take control of your health by consciously making behavioral and lifestyle choices that positively influence health outcomes. Bathing your genes in healthy habits, such as consuming diverse and nutrient-dense foods, prioritizing quality sleep and downtime, developing a regular mindful movement practice, and shifting to a gratitude mindset will be the most favorable to sustaining a migraine and disease-proof life. By changing our epigenetic autograph, we may be able to modify our genetic code to our offspring. This powerful task is at the forefront of the conscious mind: whether the passing of this genetic torch is a fire of destruction, or a fire of warmth.

Method #5: Know your Risk and Bio-hack Your DNA

Explore the following questions to better understand your DNA. What are your known genetic risks on your mother and father's side? Circle which of these conditions are present in your family history.

- Heart Disease
- Cancer (list type) _____
- Alzheimer's disease
- High blood pressure
- Stroke
- Kidney disease
- Autoimmune disease (list type) _____
- Asthma
- COPD or Chronic Bronchitis, or another lung disease

- High cholesterol
- Osteoporosis
- Obesity
- Anorexia/Bulimia
- Mental health disorders (list type) _____
- Other _____

Besides migraines, what other conditions have you been diagnosed with? What has been identified as a potential risk for you?

- Heart Disease
- Cancer (list type) (list type) _____
- Alzheimer's disease
- High blood pressure
- Stroke
- Kidney disease
- Autoimmune disease (list type) _____
- Asthma
- COPD or Chronic Bronchitis, or another lung disease
- High cholesterol
- Osteoporosis
- Obesity
- Anorexia/Bulimia
- Mental health disorders (list type) _____
- Other _____

What are your current lifestyle risks that may aggravate or activate disease risk (circle each that applies)?

- Smoking cigarettes
- Drinking alcohol
- Eating fast food
- Eating sweets or salty foods
- Eating processed foods (sausages, bologna, hot dogs, or pre-packaged foods)
- Getting less than 5 hours of sleep per day on average
- Working more than 50 hours per week
- High level of stress
- 3 or more major life changes in the last year (changing jobs, divorce, moving, major illnesses, death of a loved one)
- Unprotected sex with multiple partners
- Domestic violence
- Illicit drug use

What two words would you use to describe your health journey up until this point?

What feels overwhelming to you with regards to your health goals?

What (if anything) are you unwilling to give up?

What is one thing you can do to reduce your risk of disease?

How committed are you to making the necessary changes to reach your goals, on a scale of 0-10? (0, not committed at all, I do not need to make changes; or 10, I am fully ready and committed, I must do this).

What (or who) is your why for change?

Chapter Nine

Oxidative Stress and Dietary Supplements for Migraines

Health is a journal your body keeps about you.

-Terri Guillemets

MIGRAINEURS ARE EXPERTS IN TRIAL AND ERROR. If your response to migraines has been anything like mine, you will have tried countless pills, patches, injections, oils, devices, and drinks to cease the incessant fire in your brain. You have likely known the feeling of being let down by recommendations time and time again. I honestly had felt like I have tried it all. For my previous migraine management, I had tried anti-seizure medications, barbiturates, anxiolytics, antidepressants, triptans, blood pressure medications, and a near-attempt of the botulinum toxin injection, also known as Botox. I still have one of the newer injectable CGRP-blockers in my refrigerator that I chose not to start. Fortunately, after I was prescribed the injectable medication, I was already on my way to ridding my body of migraines and have not experienced a lingering migraine since. Now, the expired medication serves as a reminder of my healing.

Over the years, some doctors have supported natural supplements as migraine preventatives. What remained unclear to me, however, was 1) how did these supplements work, and 2) which ones should I take. No discussion occurred on the difference between bioactive forms of supplements versus inactive forms, such as which form of magnesium is better absorbed by the body. I recall taking drugstore brand supplements of magnesium, butterbur, feverfew, and Coenzyme Q10, and after having no changes in the amount or severity of migraines, I would stop taking them altogether.

It was, and still is, so important to me that I avoid loading my system with prescription medications. I do not believe healing occurs in the masking of symptoms. I respect that medications are sometimes necessary to mitigate imbalances that are beyond the body's ability. Ultimately, medications and supplements should be used to augment processes in the body, restore balance, and rid the self of suffering.

In this chapter, I will clear the air for you and give you the information on which dietary supplements are most helpful to curtail neuroinflammation, calm the nervous system, and halt premature cellular aging by reducing oxidative stress, all which are hallmarks in the presence of migraines. I will explain to you how these supplements work at the cellular level to combat cellular stress and what to look for when choosing the right supplements. Understand that we design supplements to rebalance a deficiency which you may or may not have. Supplements are broadly designed to restore balance and may or may not be in alignment with your biochemistry.

If you are taking a prescription medication for migraines, I do not recommend stopping your medication abruptly. After giving yourself at least three months of consistent practice of *The Migraine Method*, if you feel you are gaining benefits from a more holistic approach to managing migraines, consult with your physician about changes to your prescription medications. It is important to note that supplements alone will not work to stop your migraines altogether, but they potentially serve as the synergistic link to a migraine-free brain as you incorporate each of the steps of *The Migraine Method*. But first, let's peek into the cell and connect the links to aging.

Disclaimer: The products and claims made about specific products in this book have not been evaluated by the United States Food and Drug Administration and are not intended to diagnose, treat, cure or prevent disease. The information provided on this site is for informational purposes only and is not intended as a substitute for advice from your physician or other health care professional or any information contained on or in any product label or packaging. You should not use the information on this site for diagnosis or treatment of any health problem or for prescription of any medication or other treatment. You should consult with a healthcare professional before starting any diet, exercise or supplementation program, before taking any medication, or if you have or suspect you might have a health problem. The information herein is not medical advice or prescribing, but for educational purposes. You can choose how to use this educational information. Keep in mind that although nutritional supplements are not regulated by the Food and Drug Administration (FDA), it is important that you as the consumer make sure that the brand of supplements you choose complies with Good Manufacturing Practices (GMP) to ensure the highest quality and safety.

Oxidative Stress

Before we dive into the rainbow array of supplements, it is important to take a magnifying glass to the cell and examine the root reason for choosing a supplement: **oxidative stress**. Oxidative stress is the process and result of elevated levels of toxic molecules called **reactive oxygen species (ROS)**. These are the molecules that cause cellular damage in the presence of oxygen. One of the most prevalent ROS is H_2O_2, or hydrogen peroxide. Think of our cells like raw metal out in the rain, wind, and sun, subject to exposure in the elements. These various figurative environmental exposures are the ROS; and an overload of ROS causes a toxic buildup of substances that the body cannot effectively clear. This cellular "rust" causes premature aging and damages the cells in every part of the body.

Oxidative stress is the rust that erodes our cells, specifically DNA, lipids, and proteins. The inflammation that occurs because of oxidative stress can be in the form of small bursts, such as the lighting of a match, which is helpful inflammation in the presence of injury (this debris is usually cleared by the body). However, the longstanding, slow burn of a forest fire in the body is the oxidative stress and inflammation that damages and rapidly ages our cells. ROS are not just toxic substances; they are bioactive and communicate information regarding the adaptation of stress at the cellular level.

In migraines, cortical spreading depression that occurs in migraines (as mentioned in Chapter Two) can cause oxidative stress. Research shows that migraineurs have elevated levels of oxidative stress, which can further lead to the development of chronic diseases, worsening of existing diseases (such as migraines), and the premature aging of cells. One of the parts of the cell most affected by oxidative stress is the **mitochondria** – a cellular structure that plays a key role in chronic diseases like migraines. If you keep nothing else from this book, I implore you to pay close attention as we delve into the intricacies of the mitochondria.

Mitochondria: A Source of Disease or Disorder

When we eat food, there are thousands of micro-chemical reactions that occur in the body to turn that smoothie or sandwich into usable energy. In a normally functioning system that has access to balanced nutrition, this process occurs consistently, and the body converts and consumes adequate amounts of energy. When we think of energy, we generally refer to the stamina and fortitude needed to get through our tasks at work, mow the lawn, exercise, and spend time with our family. However, energy is much deeper than what we can see. The symbiotic relationship between ROS (cellular rust) and mitochondria profoundly affects the risk of migraines and chronic disease. Let's take a trip into the cell where energy is converted to see how these cellular structures affect chronic inflammatory disease.

You may know mitochondria as the "powerhouses" of the cell. Mitochondria are indeed tiny energy factories. In a series of chemical reactions called the Krebs Cycle, mitochondria, along with coenzymes, create captured and bound energy by the way of **adenotriphosphate (ATP)**. The creation of energy (by the breakdown of glucose and other nutrients in an oxygen-rich environment) produces the byproducts of carbon dioxide and water, which then releases this stored energy via ATP. ATP takes the usable form of energy to cells so that each can execute its function. Every cell in the body contains mitochondria, including cells of the brain, skin, lungs, muscles, and smooth muscle organs. We find the most abundant number of mitochondria in heart tissue, at a count of up to 5,000 mitochondria per heart cell, taking up about 40% of the space of each heart cell.

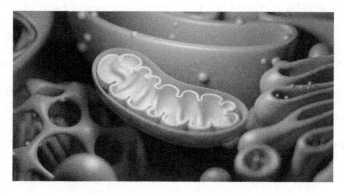

(*Mitochondria*, 2019. Getty Images.)

Our mitochondria work tirelessly to digest and produce energy for every action in our body. Just as a factory has waste products from production, mitochondria have waste products in the form of ROS, also known as free radicals. Think of free radicals just as the name suggests - aggressive wanderers seeking to destroy the things in their path. **Antioxidants** are the neutralizing opponents to free radicals. If these waste products are not cleaned up and disposed of, the free radicals damage existing mitochondria. Damaged mitochondria are not able to produce energy at the level required by the body, and for that reason, our bodies are in a constant cycle of trying to clear toxic free radicals. This is so that the body can function at optimal levels biologically, neurologically, and metabolically. Damaged mitochondria (related to oxidative stress and excessive free radicals) are referred to as the generators of disease or disorder. Let's explore this notion further.

The brain, heart, nervous system, and eyes are large energy demand centers taking up most of the body's available energy. These organs and systems become distressed when deprived of their required energy, which is why properly functioning mitochondria are so vital to our wellbeing. In chronic disease states, the mitochondria themselves are likely suffering from damage. Compare mitochondria to a peach tree - when the peach tree is healthy (roots and all), it is a beautifully designed producer of energy, resulting in healthy peaches. When the tree or roots are tired, shriveled, or damaged, however, the fruit is not thriving. We cannot expect healthy fruit from a diseased tree, just as we cannot expect to have optimally functioning mitochondria from poor lifestyle habits.

Besides lifestyle habits and chronic stress, toxic metabolites (byproducts from medications) can also damage mitochondria. Drug-induced mitochondrial dysfunction is associated with medication classes such as anti-diabetic drugs, cholesterol-lowering drugs (statins), antidepressants, anti-anxiety medications (such as serotonin antagonist and reuptake inhibitors), some antibiotics (such as fluoroquinolones), and anti-cancer drugs. Additional classes of medications that can deplete mitochondria are thyroid medications, heartburn medications, blood pressure medications, and blood thinners (Will, Shields, & Wallace, 2019). So what do mitochondria have to do with cellular aging, and why should you care about your cell's rate of aging?

Aging starts at the cellular level.

We are all aging, but we do not age at the same rate. Aging is more than a number, than aching joints, and wrinkles in the skin. Aging starts at the cellular level, in the skin cells, organ cells, as deep as in the mitochondria. Damaged or ill-functioning mitochondria speed up the aging process by contributing to a shortening of **DNA telomeres**. Telomeres are the repetitive gene sequences at the ends of DNA that are the body's aging clock. They are likened to the plastic tip coverings on the end of shoelaces; without a robust, tight, and protected end of the shoelace, over time and with "stress" it becomes frayed, loose, and unable to function properly. The more damaged a cell is by inflammation and oxidative stress, the shorter the DNA telomeres become. We associate shorter telomeres with premature biological aging. Remember, DNA is one of the codes our body responds to.

Optimizing Mitochondrial Health

It is critical to choose lifestyle habits that limit oxidative stress and promote robustly functioning mitochondria. Dysfunctional mitochondria are associated with increased nerve excitability, one of the hallmarks of migraines. Therefore, it is critical to optimize mitochondrial function for less oxidative stress. Five critical pathways to thriving mitochondria are:

1. Choosing to consume diverse foods that are considered low inflammatory and high in antioxidants.
2. Adopting and practicing regular mindful movement to keep joints, muscles, and tissues mobile and the neurological system soothed and calm.
3. Maintaining a healthy body composition to reduce physiological stress and chronic inflammation.
4. Prioritizing consistent high quality restorative sleep to remove toxins, calm the nervous system, and optimize brain health.
5. Considering supplementation with powerful antioxidants to reduce oxidative stress and premature cell aging and/or mutation.

In this next section, we will explore the fifth pathway, nutritional supplementation to optimize mitochondrial health.

Supplements to Reduce Oxidative Stress

Ubiquinol (Coenzyme Q10)

The most powerful antioxidant available today is the bioactive form of Coenzyme Q10 (CoQ10), or **ubiquinol**. This potent free-radical scavenger functions to block or lower CGRP (the main inflammatory peptide involved in migraines). The goal of taking ubiquinol is to reduce CGRP levels and reduce oxidative stress. Since approximately one-third of migraine sufferers have a deficiency in CoQ10, ubiquinol should be considered a mainstay preventative supplement for migraineurs. Studies have shown that by reestablishing CoQ10 levels, migraine sufferers can reduce headache frequency and time lost from migraines by over 50%.

It is important to take a prudent examination on what form of CoQ10 to take. Many over-the-counter supplements labeled "Coenzyme Q10" are the oxidized and less bioactive form, *ubiquinone*. On the other hand, ubiquinol is the bioactive, concentrated form that is eight times more absorbable than ubiquinone, which makes it more ready to be used by the body. If you use the economical form of CoQ10 (ubiquinone), your body must first convert it to a usable form, which means the body must do more work before it can use this potent antioxidant. This process of conversion is especially more difficult after the age of 40. Studies show that bioactive ubiquinol has a stronger effect on gene expression and is more effective at slowing cellular aging than the less active ubiquinone.

Ubiquinol is also beneficial for those with other chronic diseases such as fibromyalgia, diabetes, heart failure, or neurodegenerative diseases to restore mitochondrial function by reducing oxidative stress. To no surprise, one study showed that 70% of fibromyalgia patients have coexisting migraines or headache disorders (ubiquinol supplementation has also been shown to help ease symptoms of fibromyalgia).

Research estimates that doses of 150-300 mg per day of ubiquinol can help prevent migraine occurrence and is effective without side effects. In a January 2018 article published in *Nutritional Neuroscience*, researchers indicated that 82.6% of migraineurs who took 150 mg of ubiquinol for three months had migraine attacks drop to under 50%, compared with only 54.5% of the placebo group noting a 50% reduction. A daily dose of 400 mg of ubiquinol for twelve weeks was effective at reducing the inflammatory peptides CGRP and TNF-*a* (Dahri et al., 2018).

It is important to note that without measuring baseline levels of inflammatory markers, results of taking ubiquinol may lower these markers at different rates for different people. If an individual has severe inflammation, several chronic diseases, and only takes 100 mg a day, they may not experience the benefits as if they were to take 300 mg per day. The more inflammation that is in the body, and notably for how long the inflammation has been present, will affect how much ubiquinol is needed to clear the free radical damage and restore mitochondrial function. I found that for me, 100-200 mg of ubiquinol daily has helped the most with general body pain from fibromyalgia and has cut migraines down over 75%.

Absorption of ubiquinol can be enhanced by taking the supplement with a healthy fat-containing meal, such as with plant-based fat (coconut oil, avocado, almond butter, hemp oil). A starting dose of ubiquinol can be taken at an approximate general rule of thumb of 1-3 milligrams (mg) per kilogram (kg) of body weight per day, with higher doses of 200-300 mg total per day well-tolerated without side effects.

Estimating dose of ubiquinol based on body weight (in kg):

Adult weight in pounds / 2.2 = _____ x 1, 2, or 3 = mg of ubiquinol

Example: A 150-pound person / 2.2 = 68.18 x 1, 2, or 3 = (rounded to

nearest whole number)

68 x 1 = 68 mg of ubiquinol daily

68 x 2 = 136 mg of ubiquinol daily

68 x 3 = 204 mg of ubiquinol daily

Doses up to 1,200 mg per day have been shown to be safe without side effects, but that high of a dose is not likely to be necessary. It is best to aim for the lowest therapeutic suggested dose, between 100-300 mg per day. When looking for a brand of ubiquinol (CoQ10), it is important to look for authentic products that include the Kaneka QH seal, which is the only pure ubiquinol manufactured in the United States. Many national supplement brands contain Kaneka ubiquinol (see Resources).

Evening Primrose Oil (Latin Name: *Oenothera biennis*)

As I pointed out in earlier chapters, prostaglandins are chemical messengers that can induce pain and inflammation at the site of perceived or actual injury (such as the brain during a migraine, or uterus during menstruation). One way to reduce inflammation from prostaglandins such as IL-1β, IL-6, and TNF-a is through **evening primrose oil** supplementation. This oil is extracted from the seeds of the evening primrose plant, which is native to North America but also grows in

Europe and southern continents. As the name suggests, this plant has yellow flowers that bloom in the evening.

The abundance of essential polyunsaturated fatty acids (specifically linoleic acid and gamma linolenic acid or GLA) in evening primrose oil helps inhibit the formation of prostaglandins and cytokines by helping produce compounds that are anti-inflammatory. The omega-6 fatty acid Gamma-Linolenic Acid (GLA) facilitates suppression of the inflammatory overproduction of cytokines and helps calm inflammatory and immunologic reactions. Evening primrose oil is best known for its contribution to reduced inflammation in chronic conditions that are marked by pain and inflammation. Since one feature of migraines is inflammation, it would make sense to address inflammation at the cellular level. GLA makes up 70% of evening primrose oil, and in one study, was shown to reduce the severity, frequency and duration of migraine attacks by 86%. Evening primrose oil has also shown efficacy in moderating female hormone changes in PMS that present as breast pain, uterine cramps, headaches, mood swings, and bloating. As a bonus, GLA also helps prevent the development of plaque in the arteries by reducing low-density lipoprotein (LDL) cholesterol.

This rich oil can be effective in calming inflammatory skin conditions such as eczema, psoriasis, rosacea, or acne. Evening primrose oil helps strengthen the layers of the skin, supports regeneration of skin cells, improves the texture and smoothness of the skin, and balances water loss through the skin, all which supports supple, calm skin (Timoszuk, Bielawska, & Skrzydlewska, 2018). In my personal experience, taking

1,200-1,500 mg per day of evening primrose oil has decreased and nearly eliminated premenstrual symptoms, menstrual-related migraines, and menstrual-related acne.

Considered safe for most people, evening primrose oil can be taken with little to no side effects. The most reported mild side effect is stomach upset, especially if not taken with food. Long-term use of evening primrose oil has not been determined. It is important to note that evening primrose oil should not be taken during pregnancy, nor by those with blood clotting disorders, schizophrenia or seizure disorders, or by those taking blood thinners. Under the guidance of a physician, evening primrose oil has been used to ripen the cervix, or to induce labor.

Magnesium

It is frequently suggested that migraineurs take magnesium to help mitigate migraine attacks. But why, and how does it work? **Magnesium** (Mg) is a mineral that has an electrical charge in the body and is a vital element to all body processes. Magnesium is ubiquitous in the body, meaning it is crucial to the function of every system. It functions as a cofactor to over 300 enzymes in the body, which means it acts like a "key" to unlock biochemical processes. Calcium and magnesium work opposite to each other, like a teeter totter, to maintain homeostasis; calcium excites cells, where magnesium relaxes cells. We absorb magnesium through the gut, so an unhealthy gut may not absorb adequate levels, and an unhealthy diet may not provide enough of this elemental electrolyte. The best way to get magnesium is through food, but in many people, this is not enough to restore therapeutic magnesium levels. Foods such as spinach, pumpkin seeds, tofu, black beans, quinoa, amaranth, swiss chard, and coconut milk have some of the highest food-based sources of magnesium.

Studies have supported that migraineurs have low levels of magnesium in the brain during a migraine attack, and many also have a chronic migraine deficiency. Magnesium levels in the brain and spinal cord of migraineurs have been found to be low in between attacks. Low magnesium levels are also common during menstrual migraines. These studies indicate that magnesium deficiency may be strongly linked to migraine occurrence (Mauskop, Altura, & Altura, 2001).

Magnesium supplementation to prevent migraines is most effective in those that experience migraines with aura but is also effective in reducing other types of migraines. It is important to note that blood (serum) magnesium levels may not accurately represent total magnesium levels, since over 95% of magnesium is stored in the cell, muscles, and in bones, which is not easily measured in a simple blood test. Obvious signs and symptoms of magnesium deficiency include muscle spasms or leg and foot cramps, fatigue, numbness and tingling, tremors, depression, personality changes, high blood pressure, PMS symptoms, and irregular heart rhythms. However, with subclinical deficiencies (those that carry no associated symptoms of deficiency), a person can still be affected by low magnesium levels. For those that take triptans as a migraine treatment, studies have shown that magnesium supplementation enhanced the efficacy of that class of medications.

There are several ways that magnesium supplementation works to prevent or decrease migraine attacks:

- May prevent the electrical waves in Cortical Spreading Depression (by decreasing the excitability of nerve cells).

- Decreases and/or blocks the release of pain signaling chemicals, such as substance P and glutamate (as they stimulate the trigeminal nerve).

- May help prevent the narrowing and widening of blood vessels because of changes in serotonin levels.

There are several types of magnesium, such as magnesium oxide, magnesium sulfate, magnesium carbonate, and magnesium citrate. The following chart shows different magnesium types with corresponding characteristics and absorbability.

Type of Magnesium	Characteristics and Side Effects
magnesium oxide*	Combined with oxygen and is the main ingredient in the laxative milk of magnesia. Not typically used to treat deficiencies in magnesium and not easily absorbed. Most often in tablets or powder.
magnesium sulfate	Bound with chlorine to form a salt, most often in tablet, capsule, or ointment; most often used topically to reduce muscle tension.
magnesium carbonate*	Can be used for indigestion and heartburn or magnesium deficiency. Can result in diarrhea at higher doses.
magnesium chloride	Usually in liquid form, good bioavailability.
magnesium citrate*	Bound with citric acid, one of the most common forms, most easily absorbed, natural laxative effect, suggested to induce a state of calm. Sometimes produced from fermentation of corn dextrose, so those with corn allergies should avoid.
magnesium lactate*	Bound with lactic acid, produced in muscle cells but also found in food preservatives. More easily absorbed and tolerated in the gut and may help calm an overactive nervous system.
magnesium glutamate	Bound with glutamate, which is an excitatory neurotransmitter and may worsen migraines.
magnesium gluconate	Highest bioavailability form bound with gluconic acid, but many preparations do not contain an adequate amount per serving.

magnesium L-Threonate	Has the ability to cross the blood-brain barrier, which may help with learning and memory. Has the ability to help with neuroplasticity to form new connections in the brain.
magnesium glycinate/lysinate/taurate*	Bound with the amino acid glycine, lysine, or taurine, and less likely to cause GI upset or diarrhea. One of the higher bioavailable preparations.
magnesium malate	Bound with malic acid, which is what makes some foods tart. Has better bioavailability than magnesium citrate.

Types of magnesium suggested by the American Headache Society, the New York Headache Center, and/or the American Migraine Foundation.

Suggested magnesium doses of 300-400 mg per day, and upwards of 600 mg per day, for at least three months have shown benefits in reducing migraine occurrence, severity, and duration. One study indicated that consistent magnesium supplementation can reduce migraine severity and occurrence by over 40%. Magnesium preparations can come in tablets, powders for drinks, or gummies.

Vitamin D

Vitamin D is a fat-soluble vitamin that the liver metabolizes and converts to **calcidiol or calcifediol**, a usable form of the vitamin. Vitamin D acts as a more like a hormone and helps support nerve health and protects the body against inflammation. Researchers have connected low vitamin D levels to chronic inflammatory diseases such as autoimmune diseases, asthma, diabetes, high blood pressure, certain types of cancer, and migraines. In adequate levels, vitamin D has been shown to reduce the inflammatory peptide CGRP, which is strongly linked to migraines.

In a randomized, double-blind, placebo-controlled study reported in the *Journal of Headache and Pain*, the inflammatory peptide CGRP was significantly lowered in participants who supplemented with 2,000 IU of vitamin D for three months. At the beginning of the study, the participants had an average of eight migraine days per month. After completing the three-month supplementation of vitamin D, the average number of migraine days dropped 50% in participants receiving vitamin D. Triptan use was higher in those receiving a placebo, suggesting the continued need for a migraine abortive for those not taking vitamin D. At the end of the study, nearly 70% of the vitamin D group participants reported a greater than 70% improvement in migraines, while the placebo group reported less than a 20% improvement in their headaches. In addition, vitamin D significantly reduced CGRP levels in the group receiving the supplement, whereas CGRP levels *increased* in the placebo group (Ghorbani et al., 2020). In migraineurs, especially those with aura, supplementing with vitamin D suggests improvement in migraine severity and disability by lowering CGRP.

Studies show that **auras**, which are symptoms associated with cortical spreading depression (such as light and sound sensitivity, watery eyes, and allodynia) were reported to be higher in migraineurs that had vitamin D deficiency. Additionally, migraineurs with low vitamin D levels had reduced efficacy of prescription migraine medications. Chronic migraineurs tend to have low serum vitamin D levels. People with darker skin tend to have poorer vitamin D levels because of decreased ability to absorb vitamin D from sunlight. Symptoms of vitamin D deficiency include muscle or bone pain, fatigue, hair loss, depression, or frequent illnesses. Not everyone with low vitamin D levels will exhibit symptoms of deficiency. In one study, even those without a clinical (measurable blood test or symptomatic) deficiency were shown to have decreased migraine days after vitamin D supplementation (Hussein, Fathy, and Elkareem, 2019).

When choosing to supplement with vitamin D, it is important to know that there are two types of vitamin D. Vitamin D2 is from plants, and vitamin D3 is from sun exposure or from animal sources. Vitamin D3 increases blood levels more effectively than vitamin D2. The recommended daily allowance (RDA) for adults under age 51 is 200 IU per day, and for people ages 51 and up is 400-600 IU per day. Many migraine experts recommended 1000-2000 IU of vitamin D per day for migraine prevention. Since vitamin D is a fat-soluble vitamin, it is important to monitor blood levels with higher doses. Symptoms of toxic vitamin D levels are nausea, vomiting, frequent urination, kidney stones, or weakness. Toxicity is not common with vitamin D supplementation in adults, but it is important to consult your physician before starting.

Additional note: Although not mentioned, vitamin E is also a powerful fat-soluble antioxidant that works similarly to vitamin D to reduce oxidative stress. It has been shown to reduce migraine symptoms and prevent the need for rescue medications, especially for menstrual migraines and migraine with aura (Ziaei, Kazemnejad, and Sedighi, A, 2009).

Riboflavin and B-complex

Among the other nutritional supplement powerhouses, often recommended for migraineurs is riboflavin and/or a vitamin B-complex. **Riboflavin,** also known as **vitamin B-2,** is essential for synthesis of vitamin D. Riboflavin attacks neurological inflammation and helps equilibrate mitochondrial dysfunction. This powerful vitamin is crucial for migraineurs since it inhibits the release of glutamate (an excitatory neurotransmitter involved in migraine), working similarly to the action of topiramate (Topamax). Excess glutamate disrupts mitochondrial function, which can further exacerbate oxidative stress. Riboflavin specifically has the capability of protecting the neurovascular system and blocking a cycle of neurotoxicity by helping to eradicate oxidative stress, inflammation, excessive glutamate, homocysteine toxicity, and mitochondrial dysfunction. Conditions where B-vitamin deficiency are typically found are pregnancy, migraines, alcoholism, genetic predispositions, medication use, dietary deficiencies, and advanced age.

In a study that examined patients with bacterial infections of *staphylococcus aureus* who also had also elevated levels of inflammatory markers such as COX-2, interleukins, and TNF-*a*, riboflavin supplementation was shown to reduce these inflammatory markers. Interestingly, in a healthy gastrointestinal system, gut bacteria produce re-absorbable riboflavin in the large intestine. The more a person consumes a plant-based diet (versus animal-based foods), the more riboflavin they produce in the gut. For the benefit of a migraine preventative, the RDA of riboflavin is up to 400 mg per day for at least three months. In a placebo-controlled study reported by Schoenen, Jacquy, and Lenaerts in 1998, 59% of migraineurs who took 400 mg of riboflavin per day for three months experienced a reduction in migraine attacks by 50%, compared with only 15% of those who took a placebo.

B-complex is a comprehensive blend of B-vitamins beneficial for protecting nerves, effective nerve transmission, growth of hair and nails, production of hormones, cellular energy, and metabolism. Since B vitamins are water soluble, it is difficult and rare to develop toxicity since the excess is eliminated through the urine. B-complex vitamins include the range of B1 (thiamine), B2 (riboflavin), B3 (niacin), B5 (pantothenic acid), B6 (pyridoxine), B7 (biotin), B9 (folate), and B12 (cobalamin). These vitamins work synergistically with other vitamins and enzymes in the body to maintain robust neurological and metabolic processes, including boosting neurological energy reserve and supporting serotonin production.

Vitamin C

One of the most essential antioxidants is **vitamin C**, also known in the active form as **L-ascorbic acid (LAA)**. Vitamin C is an abundant water-soluble nutrient that also acts as an enzyme cofactor. This powerful free-radical scavenger hunts down ROS, the toxic byproducts that cause oxidative stress. Since ROS inside the cell can induce neurogenic inflammation and increase pain sensitivity, powerful antioxidants help to curtail oxidative stress and figuratively "cool down the brain" to help inhibit migraines from occurring. Vitamin C works to sweep up these ROS to further mitigate oxidative stress. To examine the role of antioxidants in migraines, one research study followed participants who were given a blend of vitamin C and pink bark extract for three months. The participants that took the vitamin C concoction reported a decrease in the number of headache days per month and a decreased severity of migraines compared to those that received a placebo (Goschorska et al., 2020).

Although the best sources of absorbable vitamin C are from food sources (such as bell peppers, kiwifruit, strawberries, papaya, citrus fruits, broccoli, tomatoes, and kale), supplementation with vitamin C can provide the extra benefits of reducing oxidative stress. High dose vitamin C is well-tolerated by most people, with oral doses ranging from 100 to 1000 mg up to three times per day. Vitamin C is a cost-effective way to help reduce oxidative stress. Vitamin C that is encapsulated into fatty layers called liposomes have more bioavailability (known as liposomal vitamin C). This form of vitamin C assists in bio delivery to the cell and gives rise to higher circulating levels than standard vitamin C.

Curcumin

Curcumin is the bright yellow substance in the spice turmeric. This plant-based polyphenol has antioxidant, anti-microbial, anti-inflammatory, and anti-cellular aging properties, and also helps keep the arteries clean of sclerotic plaque. Curcumin is a powerhouse superfood ingredient that has been shown to decrease migraine attacks and migraine frequency, duration, and severity. The mechanism of action of curcumin works by reducing the release of TNF-a in response to intracellular oxidative stress damage of the DNA. Curcumin has analgesic properties by reducing inflammatory COX1 and COX2 enzymes and reducing the expression of IL-6, which then decreases **nociceptive pain** (the type of pain in migraines). Studies have shown that enhancement of curcumin's anti-oxidative properties occurs in the presence of liposomes, which suggests that consuming curcumin with a fat-containing meal would intensify its effects.

When curcumin is co-administered with CoQ10, researchers have shown it to boost the ability to reduce the frequency and duration of migraine attacks, and the severity of associated symptoms, without side effects (Goschorska et al., 2020). Curcumin is a powerful antioxidant herb that helps promote healthy mitochondria and can ward against excess glutamate toxicity. When taking curcumin supplements, look for ones that are paired with black pepper or piperine extract, which increase absorbability. You can also cook with the spice turmeric, but it contains lower values of active curcumin than concentrated supplements.

Probiotics and Digestive Enzymes

Refer to the chapter on *Nutrition and Gut Health*.

CBD (cannabidiol)

In the wake of the 21st century, CBD (the non-psychoactive ingredient in hemp and marijuana), THC (the psychoactive component of marijuana), and medical marijuana have been widespread topics of conversation. Using the cannabis sativa plant for medicinal purposes can be traced back thousands of years, including in Chinese medicine dating back to 2700 B.C. The demand for these products has escalated for various medical conditions and for recreational use. For this book, I will focus only on non-psychoactive hemp-derived CBD, or **cannabidiol**, in the role of brain health and migraine management.

The human body contains an **endocannabinoid receptor system** present in every cell. There are receptor sites for cannabinoids in every cell of the brain and the body. Endocannabinoids play a critical role in safeguarding homeostasis by regulating systems such as the immune, nervous, metabolic, reproductive, and endocrine (hormone) systems. The endocannabinoid system has been a site of particular interest for the study of how medications and other biologicals impact this system.

Endocannabinoids (*endo*-within the body) are released in response to cell stress as a "white flag" signal to the endocannabinoid system. The endocannabinoid system (ECS) serves as a signaling system to regulate everyday body processes such as metabolism, the sensation of pain, immune function, and with migraines, activity of brain cells and neurotransmitters. Evidence also suggests that endocannabinoids play a significant role in mitochondrial health (Skaper and Di Marzo, 2012). The

ECS promotes regulation of inflammatory cytokines, helping reduce unnecessary inflammation.

There are two types of endocannabinoid receptors in the human body, **CB1** (cannabinoid 1) and **CB2** (cannabinoid 2). CB1 receptors are primarily in the central nervous system (brain and spinal cord), and can affect a person's mood, appetite, memory, pain, and movement. Signaling of CB1 receptors acts as an anxiolytic, which encourages a state of calm. CB1 endocannabinoids have the potential to reduce the over-excitability in cortical spreading depression present in migraines. Unlike THC that has CB1 receptor affinity and can induce psychoactive effects, hemp-derived CBD does not have addictive or psychoactive effects on the CB1 receptors but can induce a mild sense of calm.

CB2 receptors are primarily in the peripheral nervous system, and more directly affect the immune system, pain receptors, and inflammation of the body. During the inflammatory portion of migraines, more CB2 receptors are available for activation, suggesting the role of CB2 receptors in migraine (Leimuranta, Khiroug, and Giniatullin, 2018). Cannabinoids may serve as a cooling agent for inflammation present with one type of migraines that are specifically related to increased cytokine release.

Pain does not always signal inflammation,
but with inflammation, there is almost always pain.

The ECS also responds abruptly to **nociceptive pain**, which is pain signaling in response to noxious stimuli in the body, such as with common migraine triggers. Chronic pain can be a vicious cycle of excessive release of inflammatory molecules in response to a perceived or actual threat in the body. Cannabidiol (CBD) blocks or reduces pain of an inflammatory, nociceptive, or neuropathic nature, which are some of the most difficult types of chronic pain to treat.

Another receptor that responds to noxious stimuli such as inflammatory substances, heat, cellular damage, endocannabinoids, and neuropeptides is TRPV1 receptor, which is also known as the capsaicin receptor (the heat ingredient in cayenne pepper). Activation of this receptor triggers a flooding release of CGRP, the most potent and abounding pain modulator and the target of migraine development. In chronic pain, oversaturation of this receptor causes it to over-respond, which results in an unequal sensation of pain in relation to an actual threat. Hence, chronic pain can be a cycle against itself. CBD can block the pain signals released by the TRPV1 receptor from reaching the body, reducing the sensation of pain (Leimuranta, Khiroug, and Giniatullin, 2018). Remember, pain does not always signal inflammation; but with inflammation, there is almost always pain.

For the complex pain syndrome of migraines, studies have shown CBD to be effective at alleviating migraine symptoms at low doses. Depending on your biology, CBD may or may not help ease or prevent a migraine from occurring. I have found that with myself, family, friends, and clients of mine, CBD helps improve the severity of the migraine. More often, I notice the accompanying anxiety diminishes with use of low dose hemp CBD. Higher doses of CBD may trigger a headache, so it is important to start with low doses to see how your body responds (Meng et al., 2009).

L-Tryptophan

To expand on the mention of the neurotransmitter tryptophan in the chapter *Sleep*, **L-tryptophan** is the supplement version of this calming neurotransmitter. L-tryptophan is an essential amino acid, and acts as the precursor to serotonin and melatonin, having a direct role in regulating sleep, mood, appetite, and hormone regulation. L-Tryptophan has calming effects which can reduce feelings of anxiety and promote restful sleep. Since one theory of migraine is low serotonin, one way to balance serotonin is through oral supplementation with L-tryptophan.

In one study, researchers associated low tryptophan levels with aura symptoms such as nausea, light sensitivity, and increased head pain in migraine sufferers (Drummond, 2006). L-tryptophan supplementation can help manage the symptoms of migraines such as sleep disturbances, nausea, mood changes, and pain. Most people can tolerate 500 to 1,000 mg of L-tryptophan taken at bedtime. This supplement aids in promoting sleep, enhancing hormone regulation, and balancing a positive mood. My experience has been that L-tryptophan helps me achieve deeper sleep without morning grogginess and helps lift the mood. It is crucial to know that L-tryptophan can raise serotonin levels too high over time, or if taken with medications such as tricyclic antidepressants, MAOIs, prescription pain relievers such as tramadol and Demerol, triptans such as Zomig or Maxalt, cough syrup with dextromethorphan, or SSRIs such as Prozac or

Zoloft. As with any supplement, talk to your doctor before starting a supplement, especially if you are taking these medications.

Feverfew and Butterbur

Feverfew and **butterbur** are two herbs that have a longstanding history in traditional medicine. Feverfew, which resembles the yellow flowers of chamomile, has more recently gained traction as a migraine prophylactic, with additional claims of helping relieve menstrual pain, skin irritations, asthma, and arthritis. This herb has been used by traditional herbalists for centuries to treat fevers, henceforth its name. In a study recounted by Murphy, Heptinstall, and Mitchell in 1988, feverfew was associated with a reported 24% reduction in severity and number of migraine attacks in participants. Although feverfew is well-tolerated, some people have experienced a rise in heart rate while taking feverfew for an extended period. In those taking blood thinners or those allergic to the chamomile family, use of feverfew is discouraged.

Butterbur is a shrub found in marshy forests that derived its name from the leaves used to wrap butter. Although raw and unprocessed butterbur shrub is toxic to the liver, processed forms of the plant in supplement form have a role in migraine prevention. In a 2004 study of 245 migraineurs with and without aura, participants were treated for four months with a butterbur supplement of 50 to 75 mg. Researchers found that migraineurs found the most relief from 75 mg of butterbur twice per day and experienced a 58% reduction in migraine symptoms (Lipton et al., 2004).

ZŌK Relief (pronounced *"zook"*)

One of the beneficial attributes of targeted ads on social media is when a suggested product that you may not normally consider pops up on your news feed. During a migraine one day in 2018, I saw an advertisement for what looked like a bulb syringe used to suck out snot from a baby's nose. However, in the ad, the woman had this bulb in her ear. That day, I was experiencing a weather-related migraine related to swift changes in barometric pressure. I clicked on the link and went to a website run by a chiropractor. This small device claimed to relieve people of weather-related migraines within minutes. In haste, I ordered the device and patiently awaited its arrival.

The first time I used the *Zōk* Relief device, it did remind me of the bulb syringe I used on my babies' noses. I placed the small handheld device gently into my ear and followed the instructions. Immediately I heard and felt pressure leaving my head. My right eye watered, and within about 10 minutes the pressure left the front and side of my head. Since 2018, I have used my *Zōk* to provide relief of head discomfort due to unavoidable pressure-related changes.

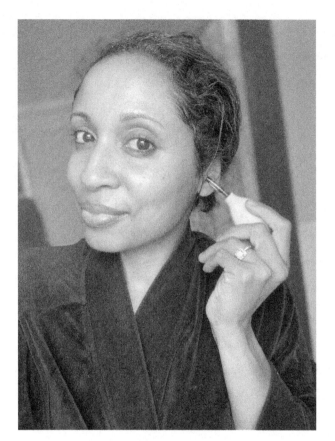

Showing the use of the Zōk.

According to the founders Dr. John Hatch and Spencer Glasgow, *Zōk* Relief works by stimulating the tympanic membrane, which enables the trigeminal nerve and several cranial nerves inside the head to recalibrate through adjusting inner-ear pressure (these nerves often overexcite due to pressure changes). This process provides instant alleviation of pressure and tension inside the head by either negative or positive pressure. This device works to alleviate symptoms that are commonly associated with sinus headaches and weather-related migraines. Since it is well-established that migraine symptoms are involved with the innervation of the trigeminal nerve, this class one FDA registered medical device gives the migraineur a rapid, non-drug method of relieving pressure from the trigeminal nerve, shrinking the migraine from the inside out.

Fertile soil maximizes the power of the seed.

Regardless of which migraine preventative you choose whether in the form of prescription medications or nutritional supplements, no pill will be effective without accompanying lifestyle changes to support balance in the body and mind. You could take every migraine preventative while not practicing healthy lifestyle habits (such as high-quality sleep, mindful movement, and positive mindset shifts), and the therapy will not work as effectively. Regular and consistent positive lifestyle changes provide the **seed** (your mind, emotions, and your soul purpose) with **fertile soil** (a sound body), which maximizes the effects of nutrition supplements and other medical treatments for migraines.

Method #6: Reduce Oxidative Stress

It is your choice on how you choose to reduce oxidative stress in your body. As stated before, x-ray vision cannot measure levels of oxidative stress, but there are diagnostic tests such as serum C-reactive protein that can give an estimate. While this blood work is not required, I do suggest that you evaluate your current health practices, your genetic risk of disease, how many years you have been under extreme stress, and what your migraine burden is (see equation below). This will help you determine your level of oxidative stress and which supplements may be most helpful.

This is for informational purposes only, not for diagnosis or treatment. Always consult your physician or healthcare provider for your specific needs.

>> Migraine Oxidative Stress Risk

How many migraine days do you experience per month? (Circle one)

1. 0-5 migraine days
2. 5-10 migraine days
3. 10-20 migraine days
4. 20+ migraine days

How many years have you experienced migraines to date?

1. 0-2 years
2. 2-5 years
3. 6-10 years
4. 11-19 years
5. 20+ years

Multiply the line number of the answers for your migraine oxidative stress risk. For example, I had 20+ migraine days (#4) for 20+ years (#5), so my migraine oxidative stress risk score is 20 (4x5=20). These scores reflect how much of a risk you may have for oxidative stress. How long you have been ill will impact your risk of chronic inflammation from oxidative stress.

Migraine Oxidative Stress Risk Scores:

- 0-3 = Lowest, 1st Level Oxidative Stress Risk
- 4-6 = 2nd Level Oxidative Stress Risk
- 7-10 = 3rd Level Oxidative Stress Risk
- 11-15 = 4th Level Oxidative Stress Risk
- 16+ = Highest, 5th Level Oxidative Stress Risk

Your score: _____

What supplements are you currently taking?

What supplements are you interested in taking for yourself to improve oxidative stress?

What is your expectation from supplements?

Chapter Ten

Yoga, Meditation, and Breath
The Bridge Between the Upstairs and Downstairs

The body is your temple. Keep it pure and clean for the soul to reside in.
-B.K.S. Iyengar

AS A CHILD I WAS COMPELLED TO BELIEVE THAT YOGA WAS DEVIL WORSHIPPING. I was around 15 years old when I first heard of yoga at all; and had believed that the practice was demonic or "new age". My parents were Jehovah's Witnesses when I was a child, so I grew up with a strict, unilateral viewpoint of the world. However, this religious identification gave me my foundational spiritual belief in God. Yet, my inner self questioned my existence and the magnanimity of the universe, and I knew there was more to my physical body and mind. "Where did my mind come from? Who is God? Why am I here on the Earth?" These existential questions coupled with a trauma-drizzled first 25 years led me to seek relief for lingering anxiety, depression, and insomnia. It was the practice of yoga that facilitated further release of migraines.

I am dedicating this chapter to the discussion of yoga because it has truly improved my ability to navigate life. Whether you yourself are open to the practice, against the practice, or a lifelong yogi, I honor where you are. I encourage you to keep an open mind and take from this chapter what serves you. Yoga is more than just a series of twisted poses for the incredibly fit and flexible; it is the art of mindful movement. If you are breathing, you are free to practice yoga. The term yoga may not sit comfortably with you, and that's perfectly fine - I encourage you to replace the word yoga with mindful, breath-centered movement. No matter what you call it, the reality is that changing the way you breathe and move can drastically improve your migraine experience and quality of life.

Yoga is not just exercise, and yoga is not religion.

What is Yoga?

Yoga is said to have originated in India over 5,000 years ago as a practice of physical movement, self-regulation, breath awareness, ethical and moral direction, spirituality, and alignment with life purpose. The word **yoga** is translated from the ancient language of Sanskrit to mean "union" or "yoke." The "union" is open to interpretation; it can represent union with body, mind, and spirit, union with breath, union between self and others, or union with God or a Higher Power. Sanskrit, which is the oldest documented Indo-European language, is often used in Hindu and Buddhist philosophies and teachings. Yoga is not just exercise, and yoga is not religion. Yoga is a practice of self-discipline, control and emptying of the mind and the senses, and a balancing union of the mind, body, soul, and spirit, the whole person.

Patanjali, one of the oldest sages in India, penned the *Yoga Sutras*, a Sanskrit teaching which became the foundation for yoga in both the Eastern and Western worlds. In Patanjali's writings, he developed the **Eight Limbs of Yoga**, which built the foundations of yoga philosophy.

The Eight Limbs are:
1. Yamas (abstinences, ethics, and relationship with others),
2. Niyamas (observances, control, and morals with self),
3. Asanas (yoga poses/postures),
4. Pranayama (breath control and life energy),
5. Pratyahara (withdrawal of the senses or separating from toxic practices),
6. Dharana (concentration and focus),
7. Dhyana (meditation),
8. Samadhi (absorption, a state of rest and wholeness, the final stage of when union is achieved).

Yoga philosophy teaches one to adopt an aimed observation of their current experience that is emotionally neutral, which includes the pain experience. Yoga goes far beyond flexible poses and comfortable clothing; it is a deeply nourishing experience that encompasses the entire essence of a person in mind, body, and spirit.

My Journey With Yoga

I am not sure what events or thought processes led me to attend my first yoga class, but I do remember it was when I was in nursing school. I remember entering this barn-turned-wellness studio and being surrounded by calm yet enthusiastic strangers. As a multicultural woman with wild hair and "healthy" hips, I didn't feel like I fit the mold of what I thought a stereotypical Western yogi embodied. I wasn't rail thin with porcelain skin, long hair, Gumby-like flexibility, and $90 yoga pants. Keep in mind, I had no experience with the yoga world except through what I had seen in the media. I did not consider myself to be physically or emotionally flexible, and I was operating more in a monkey mind rather than a calm, focused mind.

So here I was, in a dimly lit room in the upper level of a barn for my first yoga class. I didn't know yoga etiquette, such as shutting off your phone and taking off your socks. I didn't know where to find the yoga mats in the room, and I didn't understand the purpose of a block or strap. Comparable to many new yogis, I speculated that yoga was just a luxuriant workout class. My first instructor was a statuesque, thin-framed woman with a soft voice that welcomed me into class. As I looked around the room, I was the only one of my "kind", and even though that precipice historically made me feel isolated, that night I felt more connected to the other five women in the room. We were of varying ages, sizes, shapes, and personalities.

I wish I could tell you what transpired in my first yoga class, but here is the embarrassing part. The only thing I remember from that entire class is being woken up by the instructor ten minutes after everyone else had left. I felt as if someone had slipped me a sedative. Was this what it meant to fully relax? After I gathered up my courage and swallowed my prideful embarrassment, I thanked the instructor for whatever she did to make me feel so exceptionally calm.

I had fallen asleep in my first yoga class, and when I awoke, I felt as if someone had slipped me a sedative.

In the 15 years that followed my first yoga experience, I tried classes here and there. I tried hot yoga, hatha yoga, and vinyasa yoga, practicing an impressive three times a year. I always felt better after practicing any form of yoga, but even after my nervous system shut down in 2017, I still had not made the practice a regular part of my lifestyle. It was one of my coworkers who finally convinced me to make a more permanent change; she invited me over to her house one day for tea in the morning prior to our workday. We started discussing "life", and I shared how I was struggling with severe anxiety. I told her how anxiety was so prescribed that every morning as I got ready for work, by the time I was putting on my mascara my hands would be trembling, my heart rate would be above 130 beats per minute, my chest would be tight, and my breathing would become shallow and rapid. I knew why I was experiencing this methodical anxiety (reference to the chapter *Stress and Emotions*), but I felt powerless in the ability to change my circumstances.

Upon sharing all of this with my coworker, she invited me to do a meditation with her a few mornings a week at her house 30 minutes before work. I will never forget the first time I sat in her meditation room filled with colorful crystals, earthy sage, and dimly lit candles. I sat down on the meditation cushion and immediately felt like a wild bouncy ball in a gymnasium; every one of my nerve cells seemed to fire, scattered thoughts bounced around my mind, and I felt as if my body had not been that still since I was in the womb. How was I supposed to sit still in my mind and body if I was feeling restless, anxious, and uncomfortable?

I continued this meditation practice off and on for a few months with my coworker. After about two months, I started on what I call my *sole and soul journey of purpose.* In December 2018, I spent a full month in prayer, fasting (of social media, not food), meditation, and journaling. I knew there was something greater stirring inside of me. After months of journaling, reading, meditation, and weeding out things and people that were not nourishing to me, I found yoga again. I committed to spending a full year studying yoga philosophy and practicing yoga daily. As a natural progression, I went through formal training to become a Registered Yoga Teacher and expanded my practice to teaching yoga in late 2019. Yoga is now synonymous with my life, and I do not exist without it.

The Science of Yoga and Mindful Movement

The mental, emotional, physical, and spiritual skills and discipline learned in yoga can help alter a one's experience and relationship with pain. Yoga allows a person to create within their body a practice of physical fitness (through mindful movement and mobility), self-regulation (balancing emotions, stress, resilience, eating, etc.), awareness (meta-cognition, healthy behaviors, attention, concentration), and spirituality (existentialism or a deeper connection with nature, God, or a Higher Power). As migraineurs, we understand that it only takes one stressful event or shift in emotions to trigger a migraine. Yoga is an incredible stress mitigator and can help to combat some of those stress-related triggers. In the search for how yoga affects health outcomes, research has indicated that regular mindful movement practice can:

- regulate and balance hormones (such as cortisol, melatonin, dopamine, GABA, estrogen, etc.)
- decrease the perception of stress, pain, and anxiety
- improve feelings of well-being (McCall, 2013).

These combined benefits help the person amend their experience with pain and reduce their perception of the pain experience. Regular yoga practice specifically improves serotonin levels elevating the mood and outlook (glass half-full versus glass half-empty). In addition, even just one hour of yoga before bedtime can help equalize brain waves, inducing natural production of melatonin and GABA (hormones responsible for sleep and a calm mood) to promote restorative sleep.

Pranayama

One of the eight "limbs" or principles of yoga is **pranayama**, which is the life-moving energy through the body by way of the breath. It involves practicing breathwork techniques in order to master control of the mind and body. Pranayama can instigate positive, measurable changes in the respiratory and nervous system. Regular pranayama practice helps the person control their breath in times of stress, which can quickly activate the parasympathetic nervous system via the vagus nerve, prompting a path to resilience.

One of the foundational types of pranayama is **yogic breathing**, which uses the diaphragm as the primary power source of the breath instead of the muscles of the chest, neck, and ribs. Starting the breath from the **diaphragm** (a slender dome-shaped sheet of muscle that partitions the lower chest and the top of the abdomen) activates the vagus nerve, specifically during prolonged exhalation. When the diaphragm contracts and flattens, a breath is taken in through the process of **inspiration**. During **exhalation**, we release the breath out and the diaphragm returns to a passive, relaxed state. During periods of stress, tension, anxiety, or just everyday life, we tend to breathe shallowly from the top of the lungs, and the oxygen does not adequately reach the areas of gas exchange, which can put a strain on our heart and nervous system.

Yoga is the intentional calming of the fluctuations of the mind.
-Patanjali

The vagus nerve serves as the main neural highway responsible for creating a state of calm. This wandering nerve travels through the soft palate of the mouth, runs down the throat into the pharynx and larynx, enters the trachea (airway), traverses the bronchi of the lungs, provides rhythm and sensation of the heart, and finally leads into the abdominal viscera (the gut). When this nerve is strengthened, healthy, viable, and easily accessible, a person is better able to control their emotions, develop a healthy gut microbiome and ease digestion, slow the heart rate, and switch the nervous system into a state of calm versus being wedged in a perpetual state of stress. Think of high vagal tone as **resilience** (the ability to recover quickly from stress). We can stimulate and tone the vagus nerve through yoga asanas and pranayama.

There are five primary ways to activate or "tone" the vagus nerve. The most accessible way to tone the vagus nerve is through focused **diaphragmatic breathing** techniques. As aforementioned, controlled, methodical, and purposeful breathing synchronizes both hemispheres of the brain, which maximizes use of both sides of the brain (left-logical and right-emotional). Synchronization of both sides of the brain can help the person stay balanced in decision-making, relationships, and creativity.

Let's try it out with this simple diaphragmatic breathing exercise called "Three Part Breath" or in Sanskrit, *Dirga Swasam Pranayama*. This breathing technique helps reduce stress and activate the vagus nerve. Research shows this breathing technique allows one to breathe in up to three times more air (prana, life energy) than with shallow, top lung breathing.

Author's note: Stop the breathing exercise if you become faint or dizzy. If you have any medical concerns, talk with your doctor before practicing yoga or breathing exercises.

Three-Part Breath Exercise

Check your breathing right now. Are you breathing shallowly from the top of your lungs near the collarbone? Where does your breath start? Are your shoulders hugged up tightly towards your ears? Drop and relax your shoulders. Is your tongue on the roof of your mouth? Allow your tongue to fall gently and rest softly, creating a space between the teeth. Is there tension in your jaw, lips, neck, or between your eyes? Relax the muscles of your face, as if you were expressionless. Exhale all your air.

On your next inhale, start the inhalation of breath through the nose, opening the space between the lower ribs and belly button. Imagine this space filling up with air and moving upwards towards the lower ribs, then middle of the chest, wrapping around the heart, and cresting at the notch between the shoulder and the collarbone. Allow a slow and controlled inhalation lasting for a count of at least four seconds. Pause at the top of the breath, and then slowly release the breath through the nose for at least a count of five, ending with the belly falling naturally inward, towards the spine. Continue this at your own controlled pace for at least six to ten breath cycles.

The four remaining ways to activate the vagus nerve are coincidentally in the same areas of the body that the nerve wanders through. The second method to activate the vagus nerve is through **humming**. Innervation of the vocal cords are via the vagus nerve, so humming stimulates the nerve by mechanical vibration. One simple way to do this is to hum a familiar song such as "Happy Birthday," your favorite tune, or a constant note. In the yoga world, this is one method used when saying or chanting the sound "OM" (pronounced ohm or "ah-oo-um"). OM is a primordial sacred sound, representing the consciousness of self and the divine universe, and shares three primary characteristics: creation, preservation, and liberation. OM is the only sound that can be made with the mouth open (oh/ah) and with the mouth closed (hm/mm). In neuroimaging studies, the thalamus and other limbic (emotional) structures of the brain, such as the insula (that are overactive in a migraine), have shown a decrease in activity after chanting the vibrational sound of OM.

Similar to humming, vibrating the vagus nerve through speaking or **singing** is an effective tool to calm the body and mind. Think about it; if you were frantically running from a bear in the woods, you would be yelling - not humming or singing. Singing and speaking calmly vibrates the vagus nerve and communicates to and from the brain that "all is well."

This is perhaps one reason singing in the car or shower makes us feel so vibrant.

The fourth method to toning the vagus nerve is to submerge or splash your face with cold water. Cold water, especially ice water, stimulates the vagus nerve via the **diving reflex**. This neurological reflex occurs when the brain perceives that you are underwater. All vertebral mammals have this reflex, but humans experience it most powerfully. When the face (especially the inside of the nostrils) is submerged in cold water while holding the breath for a short period, the reflex kicks in by:

- moving blood from the extremities and shunting blood to the heart and brain
- increasing oxygen to the heart and brain
- slowing the heart rate to conserve energy

Since the vagus nerve controls the heart rate, immersing the face in cold water can cause a dramatic 10-25% slowing of the heart rate by activating the vagus nerve through the parasympathetic nervous system, with a response from the trigeminal nerve. In someone who is experiencing anxiety, rage, panic, sadness, or other intense emotions, this technique can be effective for slowing the heart rate during periods of extreme emotions, or with a rapid heartbeat in anxiety. This technique helps you get out of the emotional mind and into a wise mind, helping you to problem-solve the stressor with a rational mind and state of calm alertness.

Activate the Diving Reflex

Warning: Do not attempt this if you have a heart condition, take medication, have any cardiovascular issues, or if you are vulnerable to changes in blood pressure. Consult a physician if you are unsure if this would be safe for you to try. A safer alternative may be to splash the face with cold water several times.

1. Prepare a sink or bowl with cold water; ice is optional.
2. Check your pulse for one minute, either by placing two fingers gently on the inside of the opposing thumb-side of the wrist, or with a smart watch heart rate calculator.
3. Close your eyes, take a deep breath, and calmly hold the breath.
4. Immerse your entire face into the cold water, especially the inside of the nostrils, for no more than 15-30 seconds.
5. Recheck your pulse. You may notice a drop in your pulse. (When I first attempted this exercise, my pulse went from 91 to 65 beats per minute in less than 20 seconds.)
6. Notice how you feel. You may notice that you are in a state of calm alertness. Smile and encourage a state of positivity and tranquility.

The fifth way to activate the vagus nerve and promote a state of calm is through **meditation, mindfulness, and gratitude practices**. A study in 2010 by Barbara Fredrickson and Bethany Kok found that one could achieve social and relational intimacy through promoting positive emotions such as gratitude, loving kindness, and compassion for self and others. The physiology of gratitude goes beyond the superfluous mist of the mind. Gratitude can:

- Improve the quality of sleep
- Enhance the immune system
- Naturally motivate exercise
- Encourage a positive mindset and boost happiness
- Bring us closer to those we love

Areas of the brain that are activated during pleasure and socialization can be reinforced by practicing consistent gratitude, the ultimate mind-body connection. The area of the brain that is highly receptive to gratitude practices is the prefrontal cortex, which is where the right and left hemisphere meet. The prefrontal cortex helps us connect to others via empathy and helps us self-regulate emotions and our responses to stress. When we can shift our focus from a self-focused, "woe is me" lens to a more diffused lens of appreciating the people, spaces, and energy around us, we can bring a sense of equilibrium to the space we occupy inside of our heads.

Mindfulness is remaining present in this moment, taking in the sights, sounds, colors, and other sensations around us right now. One of the best times to start a mindfulness practice is during a meal. Instead of rushing through the meal to get on to the next, take your time to connect the body sensations to the mindful moment. The practices of meditation, mindfulness, and gratitude help us more effectively cope with the effects of the difficulties of life that often precipitate a migraine. Another practical way to practice meditation is in first 60 seconds of your day, before you get out of bed. Stay tuned at the end of this chapter for a loving-kindness meditation that only takes three minutes of your time.

Asanas (Poses and Postures)

When most people think of yoga, perhaps they envision headstands, poses with arms in the air, or holding poses for an insane amount of time. While those examples are certainly part of yoga if one chooses to incorporate them, physical prowess is not at yoga's core; it is far more fitting to consider yoga a personal and respectful practice, one which helps to achieve a state of peace, oneness, and contentment in those who practice it. **Asanas**, which are the physical shapes and poses, are just one way yoga brings about this sense of contentment.

The benefits of asanas help to reduce the activation of the sympathetic (stress) nervous system, increase GABA (the calming neurotransmitter), and regulate the HPA axis to help balance the mood. Asanas essentially serve as an anti-anxiety practice. Since there is a direct connection between migraines and neurosensory systems, mindful movement can be used as a tool to decrease anxiety, enhance well-being, and activate the centers of the brain and body to induce a state of calm.

Besides the esoteric benefits of yoga, more measurable health benefits include but are not limited to these points:

- Research shows that measurable changes in a person's BMI (body mass index), waist circumference, body fat percentage, and bone density are clear in regular asana practice.

- Mindful movement practice enhances functioning of the cardiovascular system as evidenced by a decreased resting heart rate (discussed in chapter three), lowered oxygen consumption (the heart does not have to work as hard) and improved respiratory gas exchange (more available oxygen to the cells).

- With regular yoga practice, the cardiovascular system (including arteries and veins) is more toned, which stabilizes blood pressure and increases blood flow to vital organs.

- Associated with cardiac vagal tone (the stability and health of the vagus nerve and the heart) is a decreased risk of heart disease, heart attacks and stroke.

- For the structural and postural system that includes bones, muscles, and connective tissue, yoga poses help improve strength and flexibility, reduce muscle tension, and encourage fresh blood to the tissues, which can reduce fall and injury risk. A warm, lubricated, and balanced body is less prone to injuries.

The Brain on Yoga

Our brain can benefit greatly from yoga through meditation, breath work, and poses, as we have established. What this means for migraineurs is that, since migraines are deeply linked to our state of stress, we can effectively combat our pain through the practice of yoga. One of the most disheartening things I have heard a migraineur say is, "If one more person tells me to do yoga for my migraines, I am going to fling them to the moon." This speaks to the mindset of the hopeless sufferer. Yoga is not a cure-all, but the benefits of a consistent mind-body practice go far beyond the mat.

Yoga helps a person train their brain to not hyper-react to perceived threats of stress.

In more recent discussion about chronic pain, there have been references to **bottom-up** and **top-down** approaches to managing chronic diseases - especially in those of the brain or mind. "Bottom-up" approaches focus on body processes such as heart rate, breathing depth, and stress hormones, manipulating these to alter our mental processes. "Top-down" strategies focus on cognitive processes such as meditation, thoughts, and cognitive-behavioral therapy to influence our bodily function. To put these in simpler terms: bottom-up approaches *alter the mind via the body,* while top-down approaches *alter the body via the mind.* My philosophy and the methods in this book incorporate both approaches with measurable results, some of which are observable to an outsider, and some of which are observable only through the one experiencing the changes (referred to as interoception).

The benefits of mindful movement are quantifiable, meaning that we can numerically measure the changes happening within our brain and body. An example of one such measurement might be a 50 beat per minute drop in heart rate during a 30-minute meditation practice. An electroencephalogram (EEG) or a positive-electron tomography scan (PET scan) can measure and provide imagery of changes in the brain during and after yoga. After practicing yoga regularly, neuroimaging studies such as PET scans have shown decreased blood flow to the amygdala (fear-based emotional center), and increased blood flow to the prefrontal cortex (personality, decision-making, and judgement). The scans can also measure a predictive magnitude of activation of the amygdala in a person who does not practice yoga consistently. EEGs of those who regular practice yoga have shown an increase in slower brain wave patterns, which is consistent with relaxation and a state of calm. These tangible results suggest that moving mindfully and controlling the breath can help a person regulate their emotions, especially emotions such as fear, anxiety, worry, or anger.

Studies have reported that in those that practice regular mindful movement, the insula contains more dense gray matter than those that do not practice mindful movement. In imaging studies, yoga participants also show more gray matter in cortical areas responsible for pain processing and attention. A well-functioning synchronized insula helps us feel more connected and in control of our emotions, even when life throws us curve balls and our world seems unpredictable.

A sense of connection and belonging is important for a thriving life, and yoga plays an integral role in reducing social isolation when we can connect to others either virtually or in-person during yoga. Regular mindfulness practice gives us a sense of purpose, a higher calling, reinforces the need for self-care, and helps us respond to stress in balanced ways.

Alongside this quantitative data, we can also use qualitative measurements to see the benefits yoga has for our mind and body. Yoga helps a person react more rationally to perceived threats, handling stressors in a more balanced manner, and therefore reducing the risk of a stress-induced migraine.

Migraineurs are exceptionally astute at knowing when something is not right on the inside.

Interoception

Humans have developed into highly complex mammals that are not just masses of bioelectrical energy, but beings with complicated processes of perception. **Interoception**, often thought of as an additional lesser-known sense, is the "internal perception" of the state of the body. It is our ability to know what is going on in our body at any given time; for example, knowing when we are hungry or dehydrated. Migraineurs have a refined interoception when it comes to pain - we are exceptionally astute at knowing when something is not right on the inside. However, these messages can become distorted when other areas of the brain that involve pain and sensory perception are not working properly.

The insula is one of the core centers that modulate interoceptive awareness. You have no doubt used your interoceptive sense many times in past migraine episodes - close your eyes and imagine how the cells of your brain feel during a migraine. The deep yet minuscule level of fiery pain (a sensation I call "zig zag static TV") is felt differently to every migraineur and can only be fully understood by the person experiencing it. As a migraineur, we feel distinct sensations at the pre-migraine, intra-migraine, and post-migraine state that may be difficult to describe to others.

Interpreting these sensations and any painful feelings or emotions that accompany them requires the use of interoception. Therefore, it is essential that we as migraineurs have a healthy and efficient insula. Considering that yoga is an incredibly effective way to look after your insula, it can also improve your interoception, helping you connect with your bodily feelings and process pain more accurately.

Yoga and Inflammation

As we know, prolonged inflammation in the body is detrimental to our wellbeing, as it can precipitate migraine disorder and other diseases. Yoga has been shown to decrease oxidative stress, or cellular "rusting." Evidence shows inflammatory molecules such as IL-6, IL-2, and C-reactive protein decrease in the presence of a properly stimulated vagus nerve, which can be done in part by the practice of mindful breathing and movement practices such as yoga.

One study showed that the average levels of the inflammatory cytokine IL-6 was 41% higher in non-yoga or novice yoga persons as compared to people who practiced yoga regularly (Kiecolt-Glaser et al.,

2010). Since toxic emotions and chronic stress can activate cytokine production leading to chronic inflammation, yoga or mindful movement may help reduce biomarkers of inflammation below levels expected with age, lifestyle, or inflammatory-based chronic diseases such as migraines.

Yoga and Pain

Pain is a common feature of the migraine. Pain that can present itself cyclically for over six months, or pain that exceeds the normal expectation of healing, is labelled as chronic; this is commonly what is experienced by migraineurs. The episodic and erratic nature of migraines means it can be difficult for some to predict when migraines will occur, which makes chronic pain even more unbearable. Every day is spent wondering when the next cycle of pain will hit.

The pain associated with migraines varies for every person, but many migraineurs would agree that it is a pain "without definable purpose." The acute pain of childbirth, for example, or a stubbed toe, has an identifiable purpose; while it can be excruciating, there is a definable end in sight. Migraine pain, however, is non-discriminatory and diffuse. Although you could likely point to exactly where it hurts during a migraine, that area does not mean that is the area of "injury". Since pain has become an expected symptom of migraine disorder and rarely has a perpetual injurious cause, we must do our due diligence to make sure the pain is not related to injury (such as a tumor pressing on a nerve). Even so, physical abnormalities like tumors are rarely the cause of migraines. I remember convincing my neurologist to run several precautionary MRIs over the course of ten years, thinking that a tumor might be causing my pain. The completely normal results left me feeling more despair than relief, not having found something tangible to explain the intense, unrelenting pain. Now, it has been a relief to learn that there are indeed tangible birthplaces of migraine pain, many of which can be addressed through sustainable stress management and consistent mind-body practices.

In my personal practice of yoga, I have been able to bypass several migraines by identifying the ignition of the migraine and immediately getting on to my mat. Whether I focused on pranayama, asanas, mindfulness meditation, or all, I have been able to reduce the intensity or eliminate the migraine altogether. Keep in mind, I have a "yoga-trained" brain, which means I have worked consistently on training my brain and vagus nerve to respond differently than when I experienced migraines constantly. My nervous system now has a well-oiled track; my body is in a more calibrated state of homeostasis than the train wreck of a body I was living in a few years ago. Even when I have had the rare migraine try to start, none have progressed beyond a few hours, and none have surpassed a level four on my zero to ten pain scale. The last migraine I experienced was related to my menstrual cycle and I combatted it by taking a dose of magnesium, getting on my mat and practicing gentle yoga for 60 minutes, using *Nadi Shodhana Pranayama* (Alternate Nostril Breathing; see the end of this chapter), and giving myself permission to be just present. Although I was experiencing the migraine, I did not *have* the migraine. The migraine did not affect my mood and the activities of my day the way that it certainly would have in years past.

As established in Chapter One, pain is an experience unique to every individual. Yoga has a place in this realm of pain interpretation. A study reported by Villemure et al. in 2014 had subjects place their hands in cold water to examine pain thresholds. Those who practiced yoga regularly could use skills and strategies such as acceptance, observation, relaxation, or reinterpretation of the sensations, whereas those who did not practice yoga reacted to the painful experience by attempting to distract themselves or exhibiting unpleasant emotions. Long-term yoga practice is associated with an improvement in pain tolerance and interpretation. Yoga goes beyond poses and breathing; the practice helps you define who you are, expose areas of the self that need cleansing, and re-mold yourself to unite and accept a union of mind, body, and spirit. These practices help the person re-define the pain experience rather than associating it with a negative emotion and further dragging down the already burdened self.

Method #7:
Develop a Mindful Movement Practice

If you do not have a consistent go-to practice of mindful movement, I genuinely encourage you to start your mindfulness journey now. I cannot emphasize enough how much it has changed my life for the better. This is not a "cure" for migraines, but the empirical and anecdotal research is bountiful to support how a steady, everyday mindfulness practice equips us with resiliency against the barrage of stress. There is an adage that compares our quality of breathing to our quality of life. "If we breathe short and shallow, perhaps our lives will be just that… short and shallow. If our breaths are deep, deliberate, and long, perhaps our lives will also be deep, deliberate, and long."

>> Assess your body and mindfulness right now.

Are you breathing with your mouth open, or through your nose? Is your jaw tense, or are your teeth pulled apart slightly? Are your shoulders tense and pulled up towards your ears, or dropped resting neutrally? Are your feet crossed, or are they relaxed at a hip's distance apart? Do you find yourself engulfed in one task, but thinking about the next one? Multitasking takes energy away from the moment at hand, and disperses it unevenly, which reduces effectiveness and the state of the present.

>> Set an intention.

An intention, or mantra, is a word or short phrase that you will repeat mentally or verbally as you breathe. As conferred previously, *our cells are listening*. Intentions or mantras are the internal communication to our cells. The body-mind rides on an energetic wave of the breath (prana). So, as we breathe and speak internally, the cells align to the energy received.

Here are a few examples of mantras for migraines:

I am choosing to release the fire in my body and replace it with cooling energy.
I am releasing migraines to make space for healing in my body.

Although I feel _____, I am accessing the peace I possess within me.

I thank you, body, for keeping me safe and well.

I have access to infinite healing within.

I am choosing loving-kindness in all parts of my being.

Write your intention or mantra here:

>> Breathe with intention.

I have introduced you to Diaphragmatic Yogic Breathing, or Three-Part Breath, which can be done at any time when you focus in the past (depression, regret, guilt) or too far in the future (anxiety, worry). Two of the best pranayama techniques specifically for migraines or anxiety are *Ujjayi Pranayama* (Ocean Breath) or *Nadi Shodhana Pranayama* (Alternate Nostril Breathing). These breathing techniques help to tone the nervous system and infuse energetically restorative prana (life energy) into the approximate 46 miles of nerves that stretch thorough the human body. The word *nadi* in Sanskrit means "flow or path of power" and *shodhana* means "purification."

Steps for Ujjayi Pranayama

1. Wash your hands. Choose a quiet, clean space without interruption or distractions.

2. Sit in a comfortable upright position with the spine straight and lifted from tailbone to the crown of the head OR lie in a restorative pose on the back with the neck and head softly supported. Soften your facial, neck, and shoulder muscles.

3. Seal the mouth with the lips closed and breath in and out through the nose. With your mouth open, exhale the sound "HAAAH" as if you are trying to fog up a mirror.

4. Now close your mouth and attempt to make this same sound in the back of your throat, focusing first on the exhale through the nostrils. Once you have become comfortable with the ujjayi exhale, then focus on the same method with the inhale.

5. Continue for at least ten breath cycles with the eyes closed and face relaxed.

Steps for Nadi Shodhana Pranayama

1. Wash your hands. Choose a quiet, clean space without interruption or distractions.

2. Sit in a comfortable upright position with the spine straight and lifted from tailbone to the crown of the head OR lie in a restorative pose on the back with the neck and head softly supported. Soften your facial, neck, and shoulder muscles.

3. Bring your right hand to your face. Place your right thumb lightly on your right nostril. Place your right ring or pinkie finger gently over the left nostril. Rest the index and middle fingers on the forehead.

4. Gently press the right thumb onto the right nostril and breathe in slowly through the open left nostril. Lift the thumb off the right nostril and press the ring finger or pinkie into the left nostril, exhaling the breath slowly out of the left nostril.

5. Repeat step four for five breath cycles.

6. Switch hands by placing the left thumb on the left nostril and left ring or pinkie finger on the right nostril. Press the left thumb on the left nostril and take a deep breath slowly in through the right nostril. Release the left thumb and press the left ring or pinkie finger onto the right nostril and exhale the air through the left nostril. Repeat for five breath cycles.

7. After reading these instructions, close your eyes, and draw your attention to the space between your eyes. Continue with alternate nostril breathing for at least ten breath cycles.

5 Yoga Asanas (Poses) for Migraines

Always seek the advice of your physician before attempting any new movement practice. Know and stay within your own physical boundaries for safe movement.

While individual yoga poses are helpful for reducing the symptoms of a migraine, it is more beneficial to develop a daily practice for consistency with the goal of priming a migraine-free brain. Start with five minutes per day in the morning: one minute of pranayama, three minutes of poses, and one minute of quiet meditation or mindfulness. Work your way up into a practice that fits your lifestyle, with the goal of at least 30 minutes per day, four to seven days per week to maximize the benefits. If you already practice yoga, pranayama, and meditation, I encourage a continued regular practice or a deepening of your practice. See Section Four for more yoga poses and images.

Balasana (Child's Pose)

1. Come to a kneeling position on a yoga mat or soft surface.
2. Bring your big toes together. Your knees can either be directly in line with your hips, or just outside of the hip width (or edge of the yoga mat).
3. Take a deep breath in and lengthen and straighten the spine. As you exhale slowly, release the abdomen and chest towards the ground between your thighs in a controlled manner.
4. Slowly release the forehead at last, either down to a blanket, yoga block, or the floor.
5. Bring your hands to any of the following positions: in front of you, stretched out, next to your hips, hands resting comfortably on the floor, or behind you with palms up.
6. Release the tension in the face, lips, jaw, and neck.
7. Stay in this pose using Ujjayi or Three-Part Breath.
8. Slowly release the hands and on a deep inhale, slowly lift the torso back up to a seated position.

Bitilasana Marjaryasana (Cat-Cow Pose)

1. Come to an all-fours position on your knees and hands. Stack and align your shoulders, elbows, and wrists. Press the open hands wide and grip the mat with the tips of your fingers and the "L" shape of the first finger and thumbs. Hollow out the palm of the hand. Stay strong in the wrists and do not allow the weight of your upper body to fall into the wrists. Push the ground away with your hands.

2. Your knees should be directly below your hips, and the legs should be hip distance apart. The tops of the feet can be flat on the ground but engaged and pressing gently into the mat.

3. Start by taking a deep breath in through the nose. Exhale all your air through the nose slowly.

4. On the next inhale through the nose, lift the head upwards and drop the belly towards the mat. Open the chest broad across the collarbone, as if you are lifting your heart to the sky.

5. On the exhale, draw the belly up and the shoulders press away from the mat, rounding the mid-back, dropping the chin towards the chest, and looking down between the knees.

6. Continue to move in this fashion slowly and methodically for at least five to ten breath cycles.

Uttanasana (Standing Forward Fold)

1. Stand with your feet flat on the floor, hip distance apart, hands soft at your hips.

2. Bring your awareness to the entire sole of the foot, grounding down to the floor.

3. Stand straight, but not locked knees, and engage your front thighs and buttocks.

4. Tuck the pelvis slightly (this happens naturally when the glutes are engaged).

5. Take a deep breath, and exhale slowly as you fold forward from the hip joint, not from the lower back. Keep the spine straight as you lower your head towards the floor.

6. If it is within your ability, reach your hands towards the back of the ankles, the toes, or the floor. It is more important to keep a straight spine that is not rounded, than to touch the floor.

7. Continue to breathe, slowly allowing the muscles of the back of the legs to release.

8. With each breath cycle, lengthen the torso and drop the head closer to the knees.

9. Stay in this pose for 20-60 seconds, focusing on your breath.

10. When you are ready to release the pose, bring your hands back to the hips. Engage the front thighs, back of the legs, and the gluteal muscles. On a generous inhale, use these muscles to bring your torso slowly up to a standing position.

11. Keep the pelvis tucked by squeezing the gluteal muscles. Center your head over your heart, and your heart over your hips.

Adho Mukha Svanasana (Downward Facing Dog)

1. Come into an all-fours position on your hands and knees. Align the shoulders over the wrists, and the hips over the knees. The feet are in alignment with the knees, and the hips with the shoulders.

2. Plug the fingertips and the "L" shape of the hands into the mat, hollowing out the palm. Point the direction of the hands so the middle fingers are facing the corners of the mat.

3. Slightly turn the inner elbows forward (this helps to protect the shoulders).

4. Take a deep breath, and on a generous exhale, lift the hips up to the sky, starting with knees bent.

5. Slowly start to pedal the feet, allowing the back of the legs to stretch gently. Draw the heels closer to the floor. Lengthen the pelvis and draw the chest closer to the mat.

6. Focus on keeping the inner elbows facing the front of the mat. Keep the fingertips spread wide, pressing into the mat and away from the ground. Avoid collapsing into the shoulders. Broaden the shoulder blades and collarbone.

7. Focus on drawing the inner thighs up from the ankles.

8. Breathe through this posture, drawing the inhale through the nose and lengthening the exhale through the diaphragm. Stay in this pose for a minimum of 20-60 seconds.

Viparita Karani (Legs up the Wall)

1. For support, gather one or two folded blankets, a pillow, or a yoga bolster.

2. Lay your support four to twelve inches from the wall (closer if you are shorter or more flexible; farther away if you are taller or less flexible).

3. Sit next to the wall on your dominant side, hips close to the wall.

4. Slowly swing both feet up the wall, and simultaneously your head and shoulders come to the floor.

5. Come into this pose and find the space where your sit bones and pelvis are at the lowest point between you and the wall. Place the supportive material under the low back.

6. Lift your head and neck with your hands and lengthen the back of the neck. Gently place your head back on the mat. Soften your face and the muscles of your neck. You may like to place a small pillow or rolled towel under your neck for support.

7. Open your shoulder blades wide and then lay them back down on the mat.

8. Release the thigh bones and into the hip sockets, and let your belly fall closer to the ground.

9. Stay in this pose with eyes closed for at least three to fifteen minutes, focusing on slow, diaphragmatic breathing.

10. When you are ready to come out of the pose, turn over on your right side and rest for at least 30 seconds before gently coming up into an aligned seated position.

Savasana or Mrtasana (Corpse Pose)

1. Practice this pose at the end of your session, with no poses following it. The most important part of this pose is that the body is in a neutral position from head to toe.

2. Starting in a seated position. Bring the knees closer to the hips and lean back slowly on the elbows by leaning on the forearms.

3. Lift your pelvis up slightly and lengthen the legs one at a time towards the end of the mat. Focus on lengthening the legs from the hip socket to the toes. Allow the feet to turn out naturally.

4. Lift your head and neck with your hands and lengthen the back of the neck. Gently place your head back on the mat. Soften your face and the muscles of your neck. You may like to place a small pillow or rolled towel under your neck for support.

5. Open your shoulder blades wide and broaden the ribs, then lay them back down on the mat. Reach the fingertips towards the feet to lower the shoulders away from the ears. Rest the hands either on the mat or on the abdomen in a neutral and relaxed position.

6. Allow your belly to relax and fall closer to the ground.

7. Release the sense organs by letting the tongue rest away from palate, soften the muscles of the face and eyes, allow the inner corners of the mouth to fall towards the ground, part the lips slightly, release muscle tension of the neck and shoulders, let the back of the arms sink into the mat. With the eyes closed, either look up into the space between the eyebrows or down to the heart. Release the brain to the floor.

8. Stay in this pose with eyes closed for at least three to fifteen minutes, focusing on slow, diaphragmatic breathing.

9. When you are ready to come out of the pose, turn over on your right side and rest for at least 30 seconds before gently coming up into an aligned seated position.

Mindfulness Meditation

As part of your purchase of this book, I have recorded a special mindfulness meditation for migraines. You can listen to this meditation by visiting: **www.elizabethpriller.com/migrainemeditation**

Chapter Eleven

Balancing Your Ayurvedic Dosha for Migraine Prevention

The 'part' can never be well unless the whole is well.

-Plato

IN THE WESTERN WORLD, health is habitually recognized as the absence of disease. Western medicine focuses on pathology (the cause and effect of disease) and curing or managing those diseases, typically in the form of medication, surgery, or therapy. Many migraineurs are familiar with seeking treatment from this western medical model. The diametrical science to western medicine is **Ayurveda**, which is the oldest documented system of health care that originated in India over 5,000 years ago. Other systems of health care such as Traditional Chinese Medicine have been modeled from ayurvedic principles.

Ayurveda practices assert the idea that, in order to thrive in life and have a sense of vitality, health, and well-being, all parts of the self should be in harmony. Instead of looking at *dis-ease* and *dis-order* as a set of symptoms of a singular problem, the practice of Ayurveda (which is the parallel science to yoga), embodies a holistic examination of the physical, psychological, metaphysical, emotional, mental, and spiritual self. When one area of the body is imbalanced, this disequilibrium trickles down and affects every part of the self, resulting in "symptoms." The practice of Ayurveda is interpreted as the "knowledge of life" (in Sanskrit, *ayur-* life, *veda-* knowledge).

Primary Principles of Ayurveda

The main tenets of Ayurveda are predicated in the belief that at birth, there is an integration of the mind (consciousness), the body, and inner and outer energy. Those who practice Ayurveda and/or yoga emphasize the relationship between the self, a Higher Power, and nature. These symbiotic relationships help develop the person to reach a state of well-being and liberation that ends all suffering. To maintain optimal health and harmony in the body-mind which eases *suffering, dis-ease,* and *dis-order,* these seven areas should be in balance:

1. Functional systems involving energy, such as the heart, lungs, eyes, intestinal organs, and the brain (*Doshas*)

2. Digestive fire and metabolism (*Agni*)

3. Seven bodily tissues (*dhatus*) which are plasma, red blood cells, muscle, fat, bones/cartilage, bone marrow/nerve tissue/connective tissue, and male/female reproductive tissue. Any persistent imbalance in the *dhatus* presents as disease.

4. Waste production and elimination such as the kidneys, liver, and colon (*malas*)

5. Motor and sensory organs such as the eyes, mouth, ears, nose, and skin (*indriyas*)

6. The mind, thoughts, and beliefs (*manas*)

7. The soul, which is the emotional essence of being human (*atman*)

(O'Donnell, 2020)

The Five Elements

According to ayurvedic principles, the human body (as well as everything in the universe) is as a whole system with interdependent parts that is made up of five distinct elements. The important thing to remember is that, if these five elements are out of balance, they can cause disorder in the body. The five elements that make up the body are as follows:

Space (Ether), which is passive and still. Body cavities such as the lungs, colon, and bladder have space that can be filled with nourishing energy or toxic waste. The other four elements fill these spaces. The ear canals, sinus cavities, and the mouth have space that allows sound waves to ricochet and be interpreted as specific sounds or words. Space is where sound begins. Disease can be present in the absence of a filled space (such as a decrease in neurotransmitters such as in Parkinson's disease, or the absence of insulin such as in diabetes) or in the presence of filled space (such as constipation in the colon or bacteria in the bladder). The qualities of ether depend on the absence of the opposition, and ether relies on the other four elements to take "shape."

Air is moving, active, kinetic energy in the form of ether, such as a breeze on a sunny day or the breath that is used to fog a mirror. Air is also the immediate start of life, and its absence is the cessation of life. Examples of air in the body are inhalation and exhalation through the nose and mouth and into the lungs, flatulence, bloating, burping, or popping joints. Air allows movement in the body, such as with digestion, breathing, and movement of the joints. Deficient air flow can appear as depression, bradycardia (slow heart rate), shallow breathing, and too much air can present as hyperventilation, anxiety, restlessness, insomnia, or tachycardia (fast heart rate). Air can be moving, cool, light, flowing, sharp, or rough.

Fire can either be warming, such as sitting in front of a campfire or enjoying the warmth of sunshine, or it can be destructive, such as with a house fire caused by lightning. The same is true in the body. Fire in the body is present in the digestive system (such as the enzymes and acids of the stomach and small intestine), the blood (which carries warmth and oxygen to the tissues), and through metabolism (creating and burning of energy from food). Fire is made mobile by air. Too much fire in the body can present as autoimmune or inflammatory conditions such as migraines, arthritis, lupus, multiple sclerosis, gastrointestinal acid reflux, rosacea, psoriasis, or celiac disease. Qualities of the fire element can be light, hot, dry, clear, flowing, moving, or sharp.

Water makes up approximately 60-70% of the human body. The brain and heart are made up of 70-75% water, and the lungs consist of nearly

85% water. The skin contains 60-65% water, and the kidneys and muscle tissue contain nearly 80% water. Even the bones contain around 30% water. This vital life force in excess can be destructive (wet coughs, sinus drainage, diarrhea, vomiting, edema, excessive sweating) or in less amounts, drying (such as dry eyes, constipation, dry skin, dehydration, dry mouth). In nature, water can be calming (a slow-moving stream or tranquil lake), or destructive when imbalanced (flooding, droughts, monsoons). Water is expelled from the body in the form of saliva, sweat, urine, semen, and through the breath. This element can be smooth, soothing, light, heavy, stable, cool, or soft.

Earth in nature refers to anything structurally solid from the earth such as stone, dirt, trees, and the meat of animals. In the human body, the earth element is present in fat, muscle, bones, and organs. Gastrointestinal elimination contains the element of earth and can be too watery (diarrhea) or too dry (constipation). This element is heavy, thick, solid, cool, hard, dry, and strong.

The Ten Qualities of Living Things and Their Opposites that Create Balance

In the science of Ayurveda, the Law of Opposites governs the state of balance. These synchronous opposites called *gunas* are how nature keeps balance, and these opposites influence the mind and body. When you use your own interoception to self-monitor how you are feeling in your body and mind, you can use this chart to balance your energy. This is why we tend to eat hot, hearty, thick soups in the winter when it is cold, and not in the summer which is already hot and humid. In the chart on the next few pages, you will find the qualities and 10 pairs of opposites (gunas) that generate homeostasis.

Recognizing the Dosha Elements

Balance of the five elements and ten opposites is manifested in the human body in the form of unique characteristic types, or **Doshas**. In Ayurveda, there are three primary Dosha body types: *vata, pitta,* and *kapha*. A Dosha is the cumulative compound of the five elements. Think about it like three different recipes for chili: some recipes have more tomatoes, some have more beans, some have more chili powder. All three recipes are for chili, but all three vary a bit in the amount of the principal ingredient. In Ayurveda, we all are made up of all five elements, but we have a primary Dosha of one or more elements.

Cool/Cold

Eating or drinking cooling foods leave you cooler and refreshed. Activities such as swimming or a walk on a breezy day can be cooling.

Warm/Hot

Spicy or acidic foods raise heat in the body, such as coffee, tomatoes, peppers, cayenne, or lemon. Activities such as contact sports, hot yoga, or emotions such as anger or stress can heat up the body.

Slow/Dull

Thick, heavy, or rich foods can make the body or mind slow, sluggish, depressed. Fried foods, sugary foods, or high carbohydrate foods can be slowing.

Sharp/Quick

Foods that create "bite" or sharpness such as ginger, rosemary, vinegar, or spicy foods can quicken energy. Activities such as contact sports and puzzles can help keep the mind and body sharp.

Heavy

Heavy foods such as cheese, butter, breads, sweets, and milk can weigh down the body and thicken fluids in the body (phlegm, nasal congestion, sticky bowel movements). Sedentary activities such as sitting or lying down weigh down the body.

Light

Foods and drinks that are light such as tea, broth, or water-laden fruits and vegetables such as watermelon, cucumber, or spinach help move energy through the body. Activities that move energy through the body are dance, boot-camp style movements, running, aerial yoga, or tennis.

Oily

Weather and environments that are humid can produce an oily or thick feeling in the body. Healthy oils that are liquid at room temperature activate the oily quality, opposing dry. Activities such as an oil massage can activate the oily quality.

Dry

Dry environments such as indoor heat or the desert can remove moisture from the body and create a dry quality. Foods such as turmeric, beans, or tea and coffee are diuretics, and remove water from the body.

Dense

Foods that contain high fat content with moisture such as yogurt, milk, ice cream, pastries, or butter can increase density in the body. Activities such as watching a movie or reading a book can ground the body through increasing the quality of density.

Liquid

Liquids can balance density by thinning out the dense substance. An example would be water added to coconut cream, almond butter, or milk to create a thinner less dense liquid. Activities such as aerobic exercise can mobilize and thin out thick or stagnant blood in the body.

Smooth

Foods that have the qualities of smooth are soft, moist, and pliable. These substances can affect every system, including the skin. Oil massages, swimming, or eating chocolate, avocado, or banana can increase the smooth quality.

Rough

Foods that are rough require extensive digestion (both through chewing, and through digestive agni.) Raw vegetables with a high fiber content that require thorough chewing help scrub the intestines. Foods such as celery, oats, berries, or nuts and seeds have rough qualities.

Cloudy

Foods and substances that are cloudy such as milk, almond or coconut milks, or cream-based soups have cloudy qualities. Medications and alcohol increase the cloudy quality in the body and mind.

Clear

Herbal teas, fruit-infused waters, aloe vera, clove, and pepper are clear foods that balance cloudy qualities in the body. Meditation, pranayama (breathing), and mint scents can help clear the mind.

Gross/Large

When referring to the overall picture, heaviness, or entirety, gross (large) qualities are composed of all cells, tissues, and waste. An example of the grossly large quality would be the carcass of an entire animal.

Subtle/Small

The subtle quality is the microscopic or minute molecule, such as a cell, thought, or pause at the end of the breath. Quiet inward activities such as meditation, prayer, or mantras have subtle qualities.

Soft

Any substance or food that is gentle, graceful, or pliable is considered to have soft qualities. Foods can be softened by adding water and cooking them down (such as apple slices). Activities that add softness to the body are massage, tai chi, hatha yoga, soft hugs, or wearing soft clothing.

Hard

Any substance or activity that adds a stiff or dry quality to the body is considered hard. Foods such as ginger, raw vegetables, or nuts offer hardness and roughage to the body.

Unstable/Mobile

Mobile or unstable qualities are moving, dynamic, and energetic. Spicy or aromatic foods such as cayenne, turmeric, or rosemary can bring a sense of mobility in the body. Traveling, moving to another location, or running can produce a sense of mobility in the body.

Stable/Static

The quality of static or stable feels steady and safe, such as the earth element. Substances that hold water in the body (such as salt) or routines that establish rhythm produce stable qualities. Meditating or practicing yoga in the same place every time helps create a sense of grounding.

I am sure that if I asked, you would be able to tell me two-to-three early signs of a migraine in your body. This is because, as the person who knows your body most, you can tell when there is an imbalance causing symptoms of imbalance. Similarly, Dosha imbalances have early signs. Beginning symptoms of an imbalanced Dosha can present as anxiety, irritability, depressive mood, indigestion, nasal mucus or congestion, increased bloating, or gas. *Samprapti* is the Sanskrit word to describe a progressive imbalance. It would be like making chili, but instead of pouring four tablespoons of chili powder into the pot of chili, you stand over the pot and shake the chili powder into the pot for an hour. If you were to eat the chili after 15 minutes of "chili powdering," you would notice changes that indicate an imbalance of ingredients. After the full hour of continually adding chili, you would notice significant and even detrimental effects; the imbalance will have *progressed* to a harmful extent. In the body, these subtle yet progressive changes of imbalance are *samprapti*. When we listen to our bodies (through interoception) and identify these early symptoms, we can add or subtract things from our lives to rebalance the Dosha and effectively support wellbeing.

There are six stages to progressive Dosha imbalance that leads to disorder or disease, such as a migraine. These stages include:

1. A buildup of a Dosha element that causes an imbalance (for example, stress or inflammatory foods),

2. Aggravation of the Dosha imbalance (such as anxiety worsened by lack of sleep),

3. Spread of the imbalance to other systems (stress, lack of sleep, and anxiety triggering the release of inflammatory neurochemicals such as CGRP),

4. Localizing in a weak area of the body (inflammation or vascular changes in the brain),

5. Manifestation of the imbalance (pain in the head or eye, nausea, light sensitivity, visual changes), and

6. Structural changes or deterioration (tissue damage from chronic inflammatory chemicals such as cytokines, vascular changes from poor nutrition, increased risk of stroke, and other effects in the body from stress).

Symptoms of disease or disorder can be compared to the leaves of a weed. If we treat only the leaves, the weed continues to proliferate, and symptoms continue. When we address the root issue and pull the root, the symptoms (leaves) disappear. The more you recognize your specific Dosha type and intentionally practice ways to keep it balanced, the more resilient, calm, and vibrant your health will be.

I believe that the relentless migraines I experienced for over 20 years were "symptoms" of the many Dosha imbalances I ignored for years. After I worked for two years to restore equilibrium in these areas using the methods I have shared with you in this book, the migraines nearly completely disappeared. Remember what I shared earlier: *for every year that you have been ill or experiencing migraines, give yourself at least one month to recalibrate and nourish your body back into balance.* This process requires patience and consistency. I emphatically believe you will be able to reach an improved state of wellness in at least one area of your life. In this next section, you will identify what your primary Dosha type is and how to balance your Dosha for a life free from migraines. But first, let's learn about the Dosha types and what elements they represent.

Primary Dosha Types and Migraines

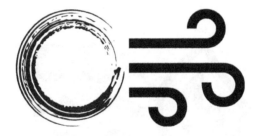

Vata (The Explorer)

Vata, translated from Sanskrit as "moving," is made up of the energy of space (ether) and air. Vata is moving energy; it helps move cells, food, and breath in the body. Emotion is *energy in motion*. Vata is calmed by the elements water or fire. When balanced, vata types are lively and enthusiastic, but are also able to easily change directions or change their mind frequently. Energy, flexibility, creativity are character traits of this ayurvedic type. A healthy vata energy promotes ease of breathing, sharp senses, healthy circulation, and regular bowel and bladder elimination.

Vatas may have a thin energized body, dry skin, cold extremities, light sleep tendencies, and thin or frizzy hair. Those with too much *vata* in the body tend to be anxious, have worrisome thoughts, burn out easily, be constipated or dehydrated, have high blood pressure, or feel fearful, isolated, or lonely. Increased vata in the body can prematurely age and wrinkle the skin. Pain is commonly precipitated by too much *vata* in the body. Migraines or headaches caused by an imbalance in vata (air) tend to be caused by unresolved stress, lack of sleep, neck tension, fear, worry, or anxiety, and are more likely to occur in the Fall.

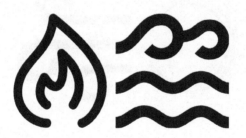

Pitta (The Trailblazer)

Pitta is the phase of transformation and governs metabolism. This Dosha is made up of the elements fire and water, known in Sanskrit as "that which digests." In Ayurveda, this Dosha helps us mentally, emotionally, and physically "digest" our experiences through fire, water, and combustion (think gastric juices). This digestive fire is called *Agni*, which is present in all Doshas, but generally higher in the pitta types.

When the pitta Dosha is balanced, the body can maintain warmth, the blood is clarified, digestion is balanced, and moods are stable. A healthy pitta balance promotes a balanced metabolism and hormones, and a supple skin complexion. A person with pitta Dosha type may be a leader or educator. They tend to have well-defined green or hazel eyes, very little or fine body hair, hair that grays early in life, a well-defined jaw, nose, or chin, medium build that is symmetrical with well-developed muscles and bones, warm skin that is prone to irritation (such as rosacea, acne, or dry skin) and perhaps either red hair or rosy cheeks and/or lips. Although pittas may enjoy a warm sunny day, they tend to overheat or exhaust easily in the heat. Pittas are soothed by water or earth.

Pitta types can be intense, fiery, and bold. Imbalanced pitta in the body can manifest as heartburn, autoimmune conditions (think fire within), nausea, strong emotions such as anger, criticism, jealousy, or obsessive thoughts, goal-oriented but with tunnel vision, fevers, or raised body temperatures during sleep. Pittas are often prone to burnout related to stress or overworking.

Migraines are commonly caused by too much pitta. Pitta migraines tend to be felt in the temples, spread to the center of the head, and are accompanied by sensory symptoms such as nausea, light sensitivity, or visual changes. Occasionally, a low-grade fever may be present with a pitta migraine. Excessive pitta (fire) migraines are commonly due to spicy or histamine-producing foods, excessive heat, dehydration, gut imbalances such as indigestion or leaky gut, anger, stress, negative mindsets, rumination, bitterness, jealousy, or unforgiveness. These types of migraines are more likely to happen in the summer but can occur year-round.

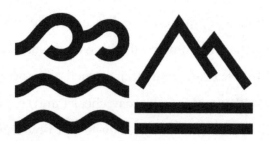

Kapha (The Connector)

Kapha Dosha is made up of the elements earth and water. As you can imagine, mixing earth (soil, rock) and water tends to result in a heavy, slow-moving, thick constitution, which is like the "glue" of the body. Kapha types tend to be consistent, patient, laid-back, and compassionate, moving through life with endurance at a lentissimo pace. A kapha body type tends to be stocky, heavy-boned, and able to gain weight easily. Kaphas tend to have moist and oily skin or hair. Kaphas are natural deep-sleepers and prefer to sleep late into the morning. This Dosha type can have slow moving digestion with low *Agni* (digestive fire). Imbalances in kapha types present as resistance to change, lethargy, depression, constipation, nasal congestion, stagnancy, stubbornness, or attachment to people or material possessions. Kaphas are balanced by fire and air.

Kapha headaches or migraines are likely to be felt as increased sinus pressure, often accompanied by watery eyes or a runny or stuffy nose. The pain in these types of headaches tends to worsen with position changes, such as when bending over. One may also notice mild facial swelling such as under the eyes. Kapha migraines are more likely to occur during the seasons of Winter and Spring.

Balancing Your Dosha for Migraine Prevention

It is important for migraine prevention to know your **primary Dosha expression** through observing yourself in different environments and situations. It is likely that while you were reading the above sections on the three Dosha types, one stood out to you as "that's me." There are seven constitutional types which are combinations of the three primary Doshas. For example, I am a *Vata-Pitta*, which is common with migraineurs. When the pitta element in your body is imbalanced, you may notice burnout, irritability, and temperature fluctuations in the body. When vata is elevated, you may notice anxiety and trouble sleeping. Once you build a solid working practice of Ayurveda, you will know exactly what to do (or eliminate) and what foods to eat more of to keep the elements balanced.

In addition to *Vata*, *Pitta*, and *Kapha*, the more specific combination types known as *prakriti* are: *Vata-Pitta* (air/space and fire), *Pitta-Kapha* (fire and earth/water), *Vata-Kapha* (space/air and earth/water), and *Tridoshic* (an even balance of all five elements). Keeping the elements pacified and balanced will help provide a stable mind and body that prevents the flare-up of migraines. It is important not to lock in your identity with a particular prakriti; instead, focus on how you can find peace and balance in all the elements. When you know what element is presenting itself as elevated or low, you will be able to care for yourself in a way that restores equilibrium. In the following section, the specific constitutions are shown with optimal daily self-care practices and seasons that help you to stay balanced. The last part of this chapter will walk you through the steps to migraine prevention through balancing your Dosha elements.

Method #8:
Routines to Balance Your Dosha

Balancing the constitutional elements in your body-mind are essential for migraine prevention. In each section, I will share with you the morning routines, foods, eating principles, mantras, breathing techniques, and mindful movement that pacifies each constitution. The first step is observing your habits, the way you respond to different foods and environments, and what makes you feel the most "well." Since like attracts like in Ayurveda, you may experience emotions and cravings that further throw your element out of whack. For example, Pittas tend to crave spicy foods when they are stressed, and Kaphas tend to want to sleep more when depressed or unmotivated.

Take a few days to reflect on these questions before you start your daily ayurvedic practices. I recommend you keep a journal of what foods you eat, what foods you crave, how you respond to weather changes, what seasons make you feel most alive. Also try to observe when you feel well, and when you don't. This quiz will help you identify your primary Dosha type.

Dosha Analysis

1. When I am stressed, I tend to react by:

    a. Feeling anxious and pacing

    b. Feeling angry, irritated, or hypercritical

    c. Feeling depressed or laying on the couch, floor, or bed

2. When I am stressed and have a craving, I tend to crave foods that are:

    a. Quick to prepare, crunchy, or dry

    b. Spicy or hot

    c. Heavy such as pizza, breads, pastas, sweets, ice cream

3. My skin is generally:

    a. Dry, light, or rough

    b. Easily reddened, burned, or irritated (such as acne, rosacea, eczema, etc.)

    c. Oily or moist

4. My hair tends to be:

    a. Thin, frizzy

    b. Early graying or falls out easily

    c. Oily, thick, or curly

5. My body type is:

    a. Thin-framed, small bones and muscles, tall, with prominent joints, difficult to gain weight

    b. Medium build, easy to lose or gain weight, supple muscle tone

    c. Heavy build, thick muscles, broad frame, gains weight easily

6. Without the aid of medications or supplements, my sleep is:

    a. Light, toss and turn frequently, easily awoken

    b. Average sound sleeper, needing less than eight hours to feel rested

    c. Heavy, I tend to sleep in late, difficult to arouse, and need more than eight hours to feel rested

7. On a 65-degree Fahrenheit day, I would likely feel:

    a. Cold, especially my hands and feet, and prefer to be in a warmer environment

    b. Warm or just right, but may prefer a cooler environment

    c. A bit too warm or easily overheated, but I do not like cold, damp days

8. My personality is generally:

    a. Lighthearted, enthusiastic, and change my mind frequently

    b. Intense, focused, and sometimes overwork

    c. Easygoing, calm, or patient

Primary Dosha Results

Number of As _____ Number of Bs_____ Number of Cs_____

If you chose mostly As - *Vata*

If you chose mostly Bs - *Pitta*

If you chose mostly Cs - *Kapha*

Your next highest scoring Dosha is your secondary type. For example, 5 As and 3 Bs would be *Vata-Pitta*. 7 Cs and 1 B would be *Kapha*, or *Pitta-Kapha*. An even spread of answers would be a *Tridoshic* constitution, the most balanced of the constitutions.

Dinacharya: Cyclic Balancing Routines to Prevent Migraines

The most harmonious expression of an Ayurvedic lifestyle is a daily routine to maximize the state of balanced health in the mind and body. The high-alert, fast-paced nature of today's world leaves us hyper-connected to electronic devices, social media, and multitasking, further disconnecting us from routine. The conceptual practice of forming routines in Sanskrit is called **Dinacharya**, which means "cyclic routine".

Dinacharya is based on cycles in nature such as sunrise, sunset, seasons, and phases of life. The ayurvedic clock encompasses the best times to awaken, eat, be most productive, and restore the body through sleep. When you move in unison with your ayurvedic clock, then you are in alignment with your natural rhythm.

There are roughly fourteen steps to the Ayurvedic routine that balance the system to prevent migraines. Keep in mind, if Ayurveda is completely new to you, choose one or two routines to focus on in the first few weeks. It can be overwhelming to make too many adjustments too quickly. Or, if you only have time for a couple of the practices, it is better to start your day with three of the steps done well than none attempted at all. The best way to find success and consistency in your daily health practice is through a concept called "habit stacking". Instead of adding more things to do in your day, pair a new habit into the same timeframe or with another habit. For example: if you rinse your mouth before breakfast, adding in the routine of oil-pulling can be done in addition to rinsing your mouth. Or, if you already have a morning routine that is working for you, challenge yourself by choosing to add in new Ayurvedic practices until they become part of your daily life. Any new habit needs to be anchored around a current habit to make it stick.

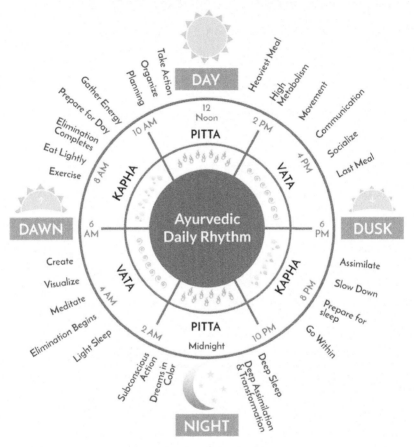

(Image from Sunshine Ayurveda, 2020)

Steps of the Ayurveda Daily Routine for a Balanced Life Free from Migraines

Step 1: Waking Up

Ideally, all Doshas should consistently wake up between 3 a.m. and 6 a.m. (known as *brahmamuhurta*, or God's Hour) when the body, mind, and external environments are the most still. The first 30 minutes of your morning set the tone for the entire day. Avoid looking at your phone, checking emails, or browsing social media in these first 30 minutes. Ayurvedic routines can take anywhere from five to 60 minutes to complete, depending on how many of the practices you implement and their combined durations. Most days, my routine takes me 20-30 minutes. Quality over quantity is more important in Ayurveda; it is more important to do five of the routines slowly, intentionally, and well, than do all of them incompletely while feeling rushed, irritated, or anxious.

Upon awakening, while your eyes are still closed, express **sincere gratitude** for at least one thing. This could be something as simple as your breath, your life, your safe space, or your ability to wake up on this day. "At this moment I am sincerely grateful for _____."

Set your intention for the day, such as an example mantra to balance your constitution:
- *Vata*: "I choose to remain grounded, warm, and calm."
- *Pitta*: "May my life reflect a calm spirit and bring happiness, kindness, and freedom to others."

- *Kapha*: "I have everything I need to be whole and move well in my body."
- Your intention:

Step 2: Cleansing the Channels

There are several channels (openings) to the body that are necessary to cleanse, prime, or nourish. Just like the oil filter in your car, we have body filters that need maintenance. Seven channels are in the upper body, which also happen to be the sensory organs involved with migraines: two eyes, two ears, two nostrils, and the mouth. The skin is the largest of the channels in the form of pores and sweat glands. The other two channels are in the lower body, the urethra and the anus. These next few steps address the cleansing of our channels.

After you arise, the next step is to eliminate wastes from the body by urinating, and if you feel the urge, eliminate the bowels also. During the night our body works diligently to detoxify wastes from the body. The longer we hold them in our body, the more toxic they can become to us.

After washing your hands, the next step is to clean and moisten the eyes. To do this, you can run cool tap water and rinse your face and eyes for five to ten seconds. Roll your eyes around to start to awaken the energy in the eyes. Use lubricating eye drops if your eyes are particularly dry. This is also a great opportunity to splash cold water on the face for ten seconds (or if it is safe for you, utilize the diving reflex technique) to awaken the senses.

Next, you will want to scrape your tongue from back to front three to six times with either a steel or copper tongue scraper, or in a pinch, a strip of floss. Tongue scraping helps to rid the mouth of bacteria. Spit into the sink and rinse the sink. Do not scrape your tongue at any other time of the day.

Oil pulling (*gandush*) is an ancient technique that is used to detoxify and moisturize the oral tissues. Hold in your mouth a tablespoon of sesame or coconut oil, swishing it around the tongue, teeth, and gums. Start with one minute and work your way up to 15-20 minutes. You can practice oil pulling while you are doing other parts of the ayurvedic routine. Following oil pulling, drink a warm or hot beverage such as lemon water to help continue the detoxifying process. Drinking warm lemon water with ginger also helps stimulate digestion and can reduce nausea. Afterwards, you may brush your teeth with an ayurvedic* tooth paste or powder.

(See Resources in the back of the book for a brand that has a full array of ayurvedic products.)

Dry brushing (best for kapha) and **oil massage** (called *abhyanga*) are two of the most beneficial practices to lovingly nourish the body and build resiliency of the nervous system. All constitutions can benefit from oil massage, but they are especially beneficial for vata and pitta types. The ancient Vedic texts articulate those individuals who practice a daily oil massage tend to age slower and are more resistant to diseases and exhaustion. Oil massage can help detoxify the skin, induce restful sleep, reduce pain, and improve relaxation, all of which are important for preventing migraines. The best time to do an oil massage is within the first or last 30 minutes of your day. Oil massage should be performed daily, or at minimum once per week if daily practice is not feasible yet. Do not oil massage on days of heavy menstruation, when you have elevated kapha (such as mucus or congestion), or when the weather is humid. Dry brushing is better suited for times of excessive moisture in the body or environment.

It is important that your energy and intent is pure when self-massaging your body. Do not rush this process. Our hands are channels of energy (think about when you grab your head when it hurts, or your knee if you fall), so you want to make sure to invite positive, healing energy into your body. Take this opportunity to care for yourself and show self-love in a methodical, caring way.

1. Warm approximately ¼ cup of clarified oil in a sink or a bowl of hot water. The best oils are sesame (warming), sunflower (neutral), coconut (cooling), or herbal oil preparations.

2. Start by putting about a tablespoon of the oil in your hand and apply it to the crown of your head (this step can be done on "hair wash days" if you are like me and do not wash your hair daily). Next, apply the oil to the face and make circular motions, oiling the nostrils, inside and outside of the ears, the temples, neck, chest, and shoulders. Take your time in these areas since they are common "migraine hot spots." Pay close attention to any areas of tension or pain, giving yourself long, downward strokes towards the heart. Apply the oil in long strokes from the outermost

portions of the body towards the heart. The abdomen, chest (including the breasts for women) should be massaged in a clockwise motion. Focus on a steady, slow breathing pattern during the massage.

3. When you are finished with the oil massage, lie down in a quiet space for about 10-15 minutes. If you are chilly, cover up with blankets or towels**. You can also lie down in a warm bath (just be careful, oil is slippery!) I recommend skipping oil on the soles of the feet before showering. You can oil the feet before you climb into bed at night. If you do not have time to lie down to rest, you can take a shower. The longer the oil remains on the skin, the stronger the benefits. **Safety note, oily towels or blankets can be a fire hazard if put directly into the dryer. Use caution.*

4. If you choose to practice dry brushing, use a natural dry brush or exfoliating gloves on dry skin. Start in the lower part of the body of the feet and ankles and work your way up with small, firm upstrokes. Wherever there are lymph nodes (armpits, groin, chest, inner thighs, neck) focus a bit more time in this area.

Nasya is an optional ayurvedic practice of oiling the nose or sinuses to improve clarity, breathing, and relieve deposited stress in the head. Full nasya is to be done only with professional guidance or the use of specialized, sterile oils; however, a modified and safer version of at-home nasya called *pratimarsha* can be done by rubbing a small amount of nasya oil into the inside of the nostrils with the tip of the little finger or a Q-tip.

The oil (often a premixed sesame oil blend) is rubbed on the inside surface of the nostrils to lubricate dry nasal passages. Ayurveda principles believe that, since the nose is the gateway to the head, nasya or pratimarsha techniques are particularly effective at addressing diseases of the head. Oiling the nostrils should be avoided if you are pregnant or have a cold, flu, sinus infection, elevated kapha (mucus buildup, excess moisture in the body), after meals, or on cloudy, rainy, or humid days. Nasya should not be performed after neti sinus rinses, as it can trap water or moisture in the nose. Nasya oil can be obtained from companies that specialize in ayurvedic products.

The optional practice of **nasal cleansing** called **neti** is helpful to irrigate and purify the nasal passages. Done properly, neti can help hydrate the sinuses and cleanse them of mucus, allergens, or debris.

1. Begin by using a medical-grade sinus rinse apparatus (which can be purchased at a drugstore or online). It is critical to *only* use sterile, distilled, or previously boiled water. Mix ¼ teaspoon of fine non-iodized salt or a pre-packaged nasal rinse salt solution in eight ounces of distilled or sterile warm water.

2. Standing in front of the sink, tilt your head slightly to the side and down, so that one ear is facing up and to the side, and one ear is down and to the side. Insert the spout of the neti pot sinus rinse apparatus into the raised nostril and begin the sinus rinse until the water flows out of the other nostril. Repeat on the second side. You may also follow the sinus rinse apparatus' manufacturer guidelines.

3. Blow your nose into tissue after completing the sinus rinse. *(Note: Do not practice neti with oil in the nose. These two practices should be done on separate days. Avoid neti rinses if you have seizure disorder, an aspiration risk, a history of facial trauma or broken facial bones, or other contraindications by your healthcare provider).*

The last of the sense organs to care for during morning routine are the ears. **Karna purana** is the practice of "oiling the ears." This practice helps to maintain the health of the ears and jaw, and headaches especially due to travel, windy cool weather, jaw tension, or overstimulation. Karna purana can be done with sesame oil that has been prepared especially for the body. Start by establishing a calm space and add 1-2 drops of warm sesame or warm ear oil into the ear. Massage the outer ear and the space below the ear lobe, jaw, chin, neck, chest, and tops of the shoulders.

Now that the physical body and sense organs are nourished, it is time to connect the body, breath, and mind through **mindful movement**. Spend anywhere from five to thirty minutes in a mindful movement practice to start your day. Below are the recommended yoga asanas (postures) and pranayama (breathing) for each Dosha type (and more poses in the Resources section).

Vata Balancing Mindful Movement

To balance vata, add qualities of grounding, peace, warmth, and stability. Imagine you are moving gently through warm honey or warm water as you practice this morning routine. Set your gaze (*drishti*) below the horizon to ground and strengthen yourself. Focus the breath on a longer inhalation.

Pitta Balancing Mindful Movement

This Dosha type needs a cooling practice that is relaxed and opens the heart and mind. Work at 50-75% of your energy level to not overexert or overheat. Keep a moderate pace, have fun, and keep this practice lighthearted with plenty of time to be free and play in your space. For pranayama, focus more on a longer exhalation. Keep the gaze at the horizon.

Kapha Balancing Mindful Movement

To create expansiveness for kapha, a mindful movement practice should incorporate space, warmth, lightness, and a bounce. After a warmup, intense movements will help to stimulate the kapha energy. There should be only brief rest periods in between poses to keep a steady flow. Keep the gaze above the horizon and sharp to elevate the energy. The breath should be controlled and with intention, so that the breath stays controlled and guides each body movement. Pause briefly between the inhalation and exhalation.

Now that your mind and body are centered, it is time to bring **nourishment** into the body. Drinking a glass of warm lemon water is beneficial to activate the digestive fire (*Agni*) and bring cleansing energy in the digestive system. Food (*ahara*) should be focused on anti-inflammatory foods that are Dosha balancing. Additional purifications of the body include drinking only purified water, using chemical-free products in the skin, and eating organic foods whenever possible. My philosophy is that if I cannot eat it, I do not put it on my body. I aim to only allow the purest to go in and on my body.

In the next few pages, I have outlined foods that are best for each Dosha, as well as additional daily practices to balance your Dosha. I recommend reading all the Dosha daily practices since we embody all elements, that way you know how to recalibrate when you feel out of whack.

Balancing Vata

Out of all the Doshas, vata is the most common to easily be out of balance due to the frequent changes of daily life. If you live in an urban area, you are more likely to have imbalanced vata than someone who lives in a rural area. Winter is the most aggravating for vata, with summer being the most soothing. If you feel out of control, anxious, isolated, or lonely, grounding yourself in stillness, warmth, and stability will help bring down excessive vata. Daily oil self-massages with warming oils such as cinnamon, bergamot, or eucalyptus in a base of sesame oil and *nasya* (oiling the inside of the nose) can warm and stabilize the moving energy of vata (refer to section on oil massage).

Those with a primary vata expression should avoid caffeine, coffee, and sugar. These substances dramatically increase the moving energy of the body, which can cause excessive vata. Foods that are warm, grounding, sweet, salty, or sour will calm the nerves such as cooked fruits, plant-based oils, pureed soups, rice, oats, quinoa, and juicy fruits and vegetables such as avocado, bananas, peaches, asparagus, sweet potatoes, and red beets. If you are not following a vegan or vegetarian diet, then meats such as chicken or fish are best for vatas. Vatas should avoid all beans except mung or black lentils. Vatas should minimize or avoid light foods such as salads, dried fruits, and raw foods, as these foods increase the movement in the gut and require more digestion.

Essential oils can be used topically (in a carrier oil such as jojoba oil) or for aromatherapy. Make sure to use caution if using essential oils topically, and always use a carrier oil or do a test patch for sensitivity. Aromatherapy is to be used to train the brain to associate a scent with a sense of calm. When you first use essential oils for aromatherapy, make sure you are in a semi-calm state or practicing mindful movement or meditation. If you only use the oils during periods of stress, the brain may associate the scent with increased stress and respond accordingly. The sense of smell is directly connected to the areas of the brain associated with memories and emotions. Give yourself a safe space to use the oils regularly in a state of calm, so when you do feel stressed, the scent may help induce relaxation. I like to put certain essential oils into the filter of my vacuum cleaner, in a sink of hot water, or on a cotton ball in my car.

Oils that balance vata are warm, sweet, calm, grounding, and strengthening. Essential oils that have these qualities are jasmine, sandalwood, cardamom, patchouli, vetiver, cinnamon, lavender, clary sage, or palo santo.

Note: It is good practice to not try new essential oils during a migraine attack, but instead try them when your nervous system is not overstimulated. If you have a known sensitivity to plant oils, avoid those oils. Do not ingest essential oils.

Balancing Pitta

Pitta is known for "moving fire" which can produce warmth, or if out of control, can produce inflammation. In general, summer (heat) aggravates pitta, and fall is more pacifying for pitta. Pittas benefit from oil massages on the head to help with relaxation. If you tend to feel angry, hypercritical, overwork, multitask, and set unrealistic expectations for yourself or others, pitta may be overactive. It is important to listen to your body, not work past the point of exhaustion, and notice cues in your body that it is time to slow down, cool off, or take a break. Pittas should strive to carve out small blocks of time for stillness.

Foods, drinks, and spices that pacify pitta should be cooling in nature and temperature, grounding, dense, and dry. Spices such as dill, saffron, coriander, turmeric, orange peel, mint, and cumin are dry and cooling for pitta. Spicy dishes, drinks with caffeine or alcohol, and sharp foods like pickles, onions, grapefruit, or vinegar should be avoided since they will strongly raise pitta, magnifying the physical and emotional heat in the body. Energetically speaking, sour tastes can even raise envy or jealousy in pitta types. Overactive pitta can lead to overeating, excessive alcohol use, emotional eating, and excessive cravings. Pittas generally have a strong metabolism and burn through food quickly. Foods that are dry, astringent, and dense are good for pittas, such as beans, lentils, chickpeas, sweet potatoes, cranberries, broccoli, and rice cakes. Grains such as rice and quinoa are dense and dry. Gentle cooling foods such as cucumbers, limes, kale, and dark chocolate provide cooling energy for pittas.

Essential oils that are cooling and drying to the body are best for balancing pitta. Oils such as jasmine, rose, mint, chamomile, and lavender help to cool the fiery energy of pitta.

Balancing Kapha

Since kapha is made up of heavy and slow-moving earth and water elements, those with excessive kapha can struggle with waking up in the morning, getting moving, or finding energy and motivation to carry out daily tasks. Developing a manageable routine is especially important for kaphas to stay focused and energized, which includes a regular work or home schedule. Routine produces a sense of predictability, which can calm the nervous system. Evening routines are just as important as morning routines and can help set the stage for a more productive day. Kaphas generally run well on 7-8 hours of sleep per night, even though the temptation to sleep longer is a common desire.

A key way to balance kapha is to introduce some sort of movement in the body every day, such as an early morning brisk walk, 15 minutes of dynamic yoga movements, or fast-faced paced exercises such as dance, tennis, or aerobics. Kaphas prefer a slow moving, steady pace versus the intense pace of vatas or pittas. However, left unrestrained, kaphas can easily fall into too much leisure, depression, or sluggishness. It is good to embrace the slow, steady nature of kapha, but not allow it to take over the day. Since like attracts like, kaphas often crave heavy, dense, oily, and carbohydrate-rich foods such as pasta, breads, pastries, pizza, red meat, cheese, ice cream, and creamy, warm, dishes. However, if these foods are consumed regularly or in excess, the kapha nature can become disproportionate and further exacerbate qualities of excess mucus in the body, sluggish digestion, emotional eating, feelings of depression, procrastination, loneliness, or lack of motivation. Foods that energize and invigorate kaphas are fresh, light, airy, dry, warming, and well-seasoned. Examples of these fiber-rich foods and spices that are good for balancing kapha are red beans, lentils, cranberries, broccoli, kale, chili peppers, turmeric, salads, fresh vegetables, stewed fruit, root vegetable soups, sauteed greens with lemon, and quinoa.

Kaphas should eat until they feel about ⅓ full, as there is a tendency to overeat which makes digestion sluggish. Kaphas should avoid foods that are sour, excessively sweet, or salty, such as vinegar, grapefruit, grapes, sour cream, milk, and processed sweets, as these foods increase water saturation in the body tissues and can aggravate blood pressure, create heaviness in the head and eyes, and predispose to obesity, diabetes, lethargy, and accelerate premature aging. Black tea and green tea are energizing alternatives to coffee, which can be too stimulating. Kaphas should drink warm or room temperature beverages instead of extremely cool or hot drinks and avoid carbonated or frozen drinks when possible.

Essential oils to help uplift the heaviness of kapha are camphor, eucalyptus, clove, juniper, peppermint, sage, lemon, grapefruit, or lavender. One of my favorite essential oil combinations to raise energy and provide clarity is lavender, peppermint, and grapefruit.

>>>

I know that I have just presented a great deal of information to you - most likely very new information - and I understand if you're feeling inundated. Just remember to take things one step at a time. I didn't become fluent in Ayurvedic practices overnight, nor did I immediately understand the principles. Identifying and aligning with your Ayurvedic type may take some time to begin with but discovering that alignment is well worth the time and effort.

If you are feeling at all unconvinced of Ayurvedic practices, remember that any positive change can influence your life for the better. These are not ideas that have been pulled out of thin air; rather, they are concepts which take a holistic and poetic approach to better understanding ourselves and our bodies. If you are open to an all-round approach to health, where symptoms are traced back to their root causes, and health issues are addressed at the core, Ayurveda may be for you. If you are not quite sure what the best approach is, but you have tried everything under the sun to escape your migraines, Ayurveda may be for you. Give it a try - implementing even just one or two Ayurvedic practices to your daily routine will benefit your mind and body.

Start where you are.
Use what you have.
Do what you can.

-Arthur Ashe

SECTION THREE

A THRIVING LIFE

Chapter Twelve

Values, Relationships, and Purpose

When there is harmony between the mind, heart and resolution,
then nothing is impossible.
-The Vedas

STRESSORS CHALLENGE THE ESSENCE OF OUR BEING. The way we interact with our internal and external worlds influences the harmony of our health. Stress injures our equilibrium, and when it is given the upper hand, we render ourselves incapable of regaining optimal health. To rebalance, there are three main approaches we can take: the aligning of our values, the nourishing of our relationships, and the awakening of our life purpose. Taking care of these three areas will grant us not only a higher quality of life, but also the resilience and stability we need to combat migraines.

Values

Values form at the core of our existence as we move through childhood into adulthood. Since values are a vital component of the self, any unwelcome change or challenge to our core values is met with resistance, often in the form of stress. If you value family, for example, you will cherish any time spent with loved ones, and you may be threatened by work schedules or life circumstances which inhibit family closeness. Another example of this value vicissitude is when we feel underappreciated or misunderstood in a personal or work relationship. What is important to you may not be important to the other person. This value mismatch leaves a gap that can cause disconnect, arguments, or even separation. We sometimes allow this bitter edge to leak into our demeanor which, at the root, is the piercing wound of a core value. Over time, as our values are threatened by people, work, school, and other responsibilities, we can become resentful, caustic, or depressed.

One of my most important values is autonomy, or my ability to act on my values and interests. I feel stressed when responsibilities exceed my capacity to maintain this sense of autonomy. When the dishes are piled high, the loads of laundry are unfolded, dinner isn't made, and the toilet is leaking - all before 10 a.m. - my day can no longer go as planned, and my autonomy is threatened. While all those things are not incredibly stressful compared to other traumas that I have experienced, those undercurrent stressors slice a laceration into my core values. Not following through with activities that align with bettering myself and honoring my values, is a huge blow to my autonomy.

Values are principles that guide our life in various circumstances. Our core values tend to change over time, depending on our life situations, stages, and responsibilities. For example, financial freedom and freedom of expression are important to my teenage daughter, and I am sure as she gets older those may stay with her. The priority of our values may shift as we move through stages of life with new challenges, goals, and experiences.

To live an authentic, satisfied life, our values should steer our decision-making. Sometimes we get stuck in a habit of saying yes to things or people that are not good for us. When attempting to identify your core values, ask yourself this question first: "At the end of the day, what is most important to me?" Some of you may answer this question with examples such as, "Work ethic, financial stability, peace, family time, integrity, courage, or self-development." As a migraineur, identifying values to steer your decision-making is of utmost importance to preserve your energy, health, and emotions. You will get a chance to identify your own values at the end of this section.

Time, energy, resources

Our core values transfer like currency into how we spend our time, our energy, and our resources. When people say they don't give a _____ (fill in the blank with a colorful word), what they are really saying is, "This is not important enough to me to give of my time, energy, or resources." Think of a situation or person that you are dealing with right now that is causing you to feel stressed. In all probability, this situation or person is draining you, because they are not in alignment with your values.

I developed a modest method of reducing stress: **preservation**. By preserving my values, time, energy, and resources when it comes to jobs, opportunities, people, events, tasks, health habits, and so on, I have been able to cull a huge amount of unnecessary stress. I encourage you to apply this simple algorithm to decision-making and see firsthand the effect it has on your migraine occurrence. *Are you ready for it?*

If it/they align with your values and it adds to your time, energy, or resources: *SAY YES.*

If it/they subtract from your time, energy, and resources, or do not align with your values: Pause, Re-evaluate, or *SAY NO.*

Use the *Time, Energy, and Resources* graph on the next page to plot the commitments, people, and events in your life that you invest into. For those activities or people that fall into the "poor" quadrant that require a significant investment of your time, energy, or resources with a low return, these are areas of your life to moderate, eliminate, or reconsider your investment. The ideal plot would require a low to moderate expenditure of energy that yields a high values-aligned return (such as autonomy, quality time, financial freedom, health, peace, etc.). The first graph shows examples of activities that use our time, energy and resources.

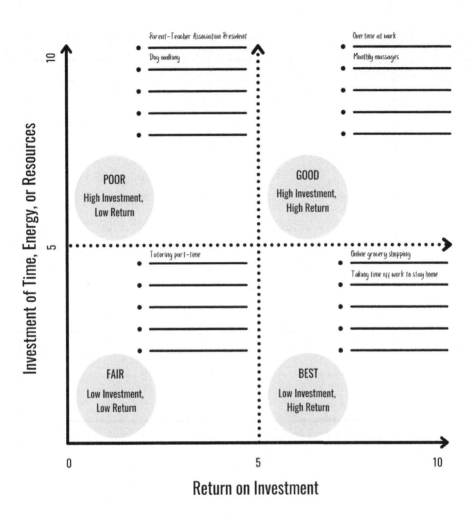

Example.

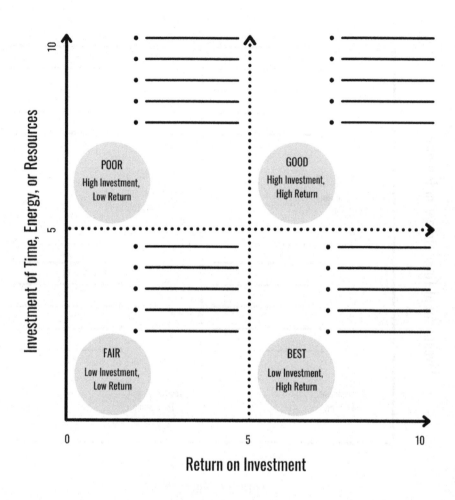

Your Time, Energy and Resources graph.

Align Your Life with Your Values

Identify a time when you have been your happiest. Why were you so happy during that time of your life? What did it feel like?

In your life right now, are you mostly in a state of having, doing, or being?

Identify a time you felt fulfilled, on track in life, or successful. What was happening during that time and why were you feeling fulfilled?

Read through this list of values on the next few pages, and then select the first 10 that stand out to you.

❏ Accountability	❏ Balance
❏ Accuracy	❏ Being the best
❏ Achievement	❏ Belonging
❏ Adventurousness	❏ Boldness
❏ Altruism	❏ Calmness
❏ Ambition	❏ Carefulness
❏ Assertiveness	❏ Challenge

- ❑ Cheerfulness
- ❑ Clear mindedness
- ❑ Commitment
- ❑ Community
- ❑ Compassion
- ❑ Competitiveness
- ❑ Consistency
- ❑ Contentment
- ❑ Continuous Improvement
- ❑ Contribution
- ❑ Control
- ❑ Cooperation
- ❑ Correctness
- ❑ Courtesy
- ❑ Creativity
- ❑ Curiosity
- ❑ Decisiveness
- ❑ Dependability
- ❑ Determination
- ❑ Devoutness
- ❑ Diligence
- ❑ Discipline
- ❑ Discretion
- ❑ Diversity
- ❑ Dynamism
- ❑ Economy
- ❑ Effectiveness
- ❑ Efficiency
- ❑ Elegance
- ❑ Empathy

- ❑ Enjoyment
- ❑ Enthusiasm
- ❑ Equality Excellence
- ❑ Excitement
- ❑ Expertise
- ❑ Exploration
- ❑ Expressiveness
- ❑ Fairness
- ❑ Faith
- ❑ Family-oriented
- ❑ Fidelity
- ❑ Fitness
- ❑ Fluency
- ❑ Focus
- ❑ Freedom
- ❑ Fun
- ❑ Generosity
- ❑ Goodness
- ❑ Grace
- ❑ Growth
- ❑ Happiness
- ❑ Hard Work
- ❑ Health
- ❑ Helping Society
- ❑ Holiness
- ❑ Honesty
- ❑ Honor
- ❑ Humility
- ❑ Independence
- ❑ Ingenuity

- ❏ Inner Harmony
- ❏ Inquisitiveness
- ❏ Insightfulness
- ❏ Intelligence
- ❏ Intellectual Status
- ❏ Intuition
- ❏ Joy
- ❏ Justice
- ❏ Leadership
- ❏ Legacy
- ❏ Love
- ❏ Loyalty
- ❏ Making a difference
- ❏ Mastery
- ❏ Merit
- ❏ Obedience
- ❏ Openness
- ❏ Order
- ❏ Originality
- ❏ Patriotism
- ❏ Perfection
- ❏ Piety
- ❏ Positivity
- ❏ Practicality
- ❏ Preparedness
- ❏ Professionalism
- ❏ Prudence
- ❏ Quality-orientation
- ❏ Reliability
- ❏ Resourcefulness
- ❏ Restraint
- ❏ Results-oriented
- ❏ Rigor
- ❏ Security
- ❏ Self-actualization
- ❏ Self-control
- ❏ Selflessness
- ❏ Self-reliance
- ❏ Sensitivity
- ❏ Serenity
- ❏ Service
- ❏ Shrewdness
- ❏ Simplicity
- ❏ Soundness
- ❏ Speed
- ❏ Spontaneity
- ❏ Stability
- ❏ Strategic
- ❏ Strength
- ❏ Structure
- ❏ Success
- ❏ Support
- ❏ Teamwork
- ❏ Temperance
- ❏ Thankfulness
- ❏ Thoroughness
- ❏ Thoughtfulness
- ❏ Timeliness
- ❏ Tolerance
- ❏ Traditionalism

❏ Trustworthiness   ❏ Usefulness

❏ Truth-seeking   ❏ Vision

❏ Understanding   ❏ Vitality

❏ Uniqueness   ❏ Other _____

❏ Unity

Out of that list of ten value-words, think about the first two scenarios of when you felt most fulfilled and happy. Which three of these words align most with those times in your life? Write those three value words here.

1. _____

2. _____

3. _____

In this current season of your life, *these are your core values*, or what is most important to you to feel fulfilled, vibrant, satisfied, and on your way to a thriving life. Now, ask yourself the following questions:

- What is the number one thing that you feel the most stressed by right now?

- Does this stressor/person/situation *align with one or all your core values,* or does it *challenge or destroy at least one of your core values?*

- Does this stressor/person/situation *steal from* or *give to* your time, energy, or resources?

- What needs to change for this stressor/person/situation to give you back some of your time, energy, or resources, or to align with your core values?

- What part of this change can you control?

- What active steps have you taken to balance your time, energy, and resources?

- How do you communicate your values to others?

As you can see, identifying your core values and using them as decision-making navigators can be challenging. If doing so will point you towards a thriving life that preserves your time, energy, and resources, I am sure you will agree that this practice is well worth the effort. As you move forward with decision-making, ask yourself if the decision/person/stressor/opportunity **adds** to your life, or **subtracts** from your life. These value-based principles will help you ease stress and tension, which contributes to migraine prevention.

Relationships

I am not a relationship expert, but I am confident that unhealthy relationships have been a troublesome root of migraines for many sufferers. Relationships are complex and ubiquitous; interacting with other humans, whether briefly at the bus stop, or in a lifelong relationship with a partner or child, is one of the most intricate aspects of human life. The connections we form with other people play a role in shaping who we are and who we will become. Solid, supportive, mutually respectful relationships are vital for our wellbeing; as social creatures, we long to connect with those who value and enrich us. A host of research supports the connection between relationships and wellbeing - it should not come as a surprise that relationships might have an impact on our mental and physical health, and by extension, our migraine experience.

The humorous quote, "You can pick your nose, but you can't pick your family," is ever accurate. Sometimes family relationships can be the most challenging, as we feel obligated to love our family, though we may not like them or feel valued by them at times. Other kinds of relationships, such as with co-workers, supervisors, physician-patient, hairdressers, landlords, acquaintances, or friends, can be challenging too; the dynamics of the relationship directly affect our mind, emotions, biology, and stress adaptation. Perhaps you have that one friend who talks incessantly about their life drama (*or perhaps you are that friend*). Maybe you interact with someone who is dominating, controlling, or hypercritical. That type of negativity will put a strain on the relationship, as neither party is being enriched or uplifted by these interactions.

Unless you are an apathetic robot, the relationships in your life will influence your mental, emotional, spiritual, and physical health in some way. For this reason, it is so important to pay attention to your energy after you spend time with someone. If you feel enlightened, happy, and energetic, that relationship is likely healthy. However, if you feel drained, depressed, anxious, or lethargic after spending time with that person, *listen to your body*. Remember, we have monitoring systems in the body (the insula, amygdala, vagus nerve, hypothalamus, to name a few) that monitor the people and situations we interact with - all to keep you safe and thriving.

This is not to say to break up with your significant other the first time he or she annoys you, or to resign your relationship with a pessimistic friend. Every relationship has conflict; every individual person brings their own challenges to a relationship. It is about reflecting on the whole relationship, assessing whether it is lifting you up or weighing you down. I do encourage you to assess, accept, and nurture the relationships you choose to have in your life - including your relationship with yourself. Focusing inward is a good place to start.

Self-worth is an inside job.

The Relationship With Self

You are the person that you have known the longest. You are the only person on the planet with full access into your inner world; the only person who sees the world from your perspective. The relationship you have with yourself is the foundation for all other relationships - if you have love and respect for yourself, you can show the same love and respect to others. While it is true that people that do not love and respect themselves can still be some of the most outwardly loving people you will ever meet, the way they interpret love in return will often be distorted. They may also struggle to maintain secure relationships as a result of not having a stable relationship with themselves. The self-love conversation can easily lead into personality and mental health disorders, but for now, let's explore healthy self-love and what it means to nurture your inner relationship.

What is your first memory? Our early memories are usually a time when an emotion was paired with an event, locking it into long-term memory. I recall one of my earliest childhood memories at my grandparent's home when I was about three years old. I had watched my grandfather shave his face with a straight razor on countless occasions, and in my naivety, I assumed that shaving the face was what everyone did. I recall one morning gathering a step stool and assembling my grandfather's shaving supplies. I lathered my face and began to run the chiseled blade across my cheeks. I remember feeling confident, moving the blades across my face in an austere manner. As you can imagine, a three-year-old girl shaving with a straight razor cannot possibly end well. Once I saw the fresh peeks of crimson running down my cheeks, I hastily blotted at my face with tissues and grabbed the first aid kit. 15 mini-Band-Aids later I emerged from the bathroom and went out into the family room as if nothing was amiss.

This early childhood memory was the first time I remember feeling aware of myself. I recall looking into the mirror and making the decision to shave my face. I remember feeling confident and curious. When I think about this event now, I can see similarities in my personality and how I view myself in the present day compared to my younger self. I consider myself a confident person with an inquisitiveness for trying new things. I am also the type of person to see someone do something and feel the need to prove that I can accomplish it just as well (such as my experiences as a volunteer firefighter, auxiliary police officer, and flying an airplane for my birthday). Your relationship with yourself has likely morphed over the years of your life, however, there are more similarities than you might realize. Who we view ourselves to be on the first day of kindergarten might be quite similar to who we view ourselves to be today.

Your relationship with migraines magnifies parts of yourself that may or may not be the parts you wish to embody. During periods of suffering, I remember pondering, *Who am I without migraines?* Outside of migraines, I am confident that I am a vibrant, passionate, empathetic, and optimistic person. However, when I was stuck in the thick cloud of migraine explosions, I became angry, bitter, pessimistic, and woeful. As soon as the migraine dust would clear, I became that energetic beam of sunshine again. Can you relate to this dichotomous personality shift? One of the reasons I believe this shift occurs (besides the neurobiological catalytic reactions in the brain) is because of how closely we identify with our pain and suffering. Just as this book started, we tend to "own" our migraines. When we are suffering, many parts of our lives are controlled by migraines. We sometimes blame our behaviors on our suffering, as if it is a pass to be sharp in the way we talk to others through the negative-focused lens we tend to see the world from. I can comfortably bring this up because I have been there (and I consciously refocus my lens daily). Countless times I have had to apologize to those closest to me for projecting my irritability and frustration of suffering during a migraine.

Mending and nurturing your relationship with yourself will require you to recognize these things; that your migraines are not a feature of your personality, nor do they define who you are. Self-relationship is also about becoming familiar with your progression from childhood to adulthood.

How did you view yourself as a child? How has your view of yourself changed since then, and what sparked that change? What parts of yourself can you empathize with, having been with yourself since birth? Reflection will be your greatest ally when mending the relationship with yourself.

Your Relationships With Others

We mirror the five people we spend the most time with. How do the people in your life influence your migraine journey? How do your closest relationships impact your values? What is your role in your family, social circle, or work group? Do these five people add to your sense of wellbeing? Do any of these five people increase stress in your body or mind, or do they distract you from fulfilling your greatest purpose? These are questions that may guide you to evaluate how your closest relationships influence your perspective about your experiences and purpose in the world.

At the most fundamental level, conflict arises in relationships due to a mismatch in values. Think of a time when you had conflict with someone. Perhaps you were trying to convey a message, and the person interpreted or received the message differently than your intent, implying that their values were threatened. You may have found yourself in a situation where a close friend acted in a way that misaligned with your values (for example, if they felt upset and responded by giving you the cold shoulder instead of being upfront and honest). When our values align with another person's values, there is less friction in the relationship. When there is a mismatch of values, tension and stress can be present in the relationship, which further escalates inner turmoil in a frayed migraine brain.

Your Relationship With A Higher Power

What do the words universe, existence, God, Divine, soul, Mother Nature, source energy, Higher Power, prayer, and meditation mean to you? Where do thoughts come from? What is our existence without memories, thoughts, and emotions? What underpins this concept of spirituality? We are free to define and interpret spirituality as it fits our belief system and greater purpose. There are many sectors of spirituality, but ultimately, spirituality refers to the human phenomenon of being drawn to something outside (or inside) of ourselves that is greater than the physical body.

> *A thick, hard, closed mind is of limited benefit.*
> *Endless difficulties arise for inflexible minds.*
> - Lama Zopa Rinpoche

The migraineur's experience with pain and suffering is deeply rooted in the individual spiritual journey. Many of us have clung to a faith in something greater than us when we are suffering; migraine sufferers may pray, meditate, hope, or scream into the universe for momentary pain relief or complete healing. Wherever you are on your journey of spirituality, I implore you to keep your mind open and elastic to how your spirituality is connected to your experience with migraines. It is essential that in your migraine journey you do not close off hope to the end of your suffering. The space where your thoughts and beliefs reside is coincidentally where most migraines are experienced: the head. Lama Zopa Rinpoche, a Buddhist master, believed that "A thick, hard, closed mind is of limited benefit; endless difficulties arise for inflexible minds."

Pruning and Fresh Beginnings

A gardener knows that pruning is an essential practice for improving the health of the plant. Humans also require pruning to encourage health and vitality of the self. This practice does not involve cutting off physical parts of the body, but instead requires pruning of relational, mental, or emotional areas that impede growth. Pruning can be a painful, disruptive process to our current expectations. To flourish, we must focus on our best parts by urgently removing parts that hinder our potential.

Pruning can be unpleasant. When I first applied the principle of pruning in my vegetable and flower garden, I was saddened to have to cut off perfectly good stems or flower buds. As a compassionate person, I never want to harm any living thing - not even a plant. I identified the plants I wanted to blossom, and then intently chopped off the stems that would suck nutrients and energy from that bloom. Sometimes I had to wait months or years before I saw the "fruit" of pruning. In the waiting season, the plant looked misshapen, bare, and veiny. This awkward phase was all worthwhile once I was patient enough to see the bountiful results.

When stems of life are dead or diseased, it can be much easier to prune to save the rest of the plant, in the same way that reaching your lowest point in life can give you the motivation to bounce back. When you feel you are doing good things, however, it becomes much more difficult deciding what to cut out of your life. What do you do when something that should be beneficial to you is dragging you down? Is it possible that something can be 'good' in and of itself, but not necessarily good for you?

We cannot heal or grow in the same place we were hurt.

I have pruned myself from committees, jobs, relationships, duties, beliefs, and practices that were draining and stunting my growth and healing. Although my previous corporate job seemed essentially 'good,' it was draining me and making me physically ill because of toxic work environments and misalignment with my values and greater purpose. I wrestled with the false belief that I had to keep pressing on; so, I dealt with unhealthy "limbs" in order to feel successful. I struggled with the false belief that perhaps I wasn't resilient enough to deal with what I was experiencing, or that this was the price I had to pay for success. The outside world saw me as successful, while I was experiencing necrotic lesions in my soul, body, and mind. After studying the teachings of Dr. Henry Cloud's book, *Necessary Endings*, I realized I had to make painful but necessary cuts in my life in order to receive what was best for me. This practice has led me to where I am today. Just as with gardening, we must continually evaluate areas that may need pruning. We cannot heal or grow in the same place we were hurt. Sometimes a healthy pruning is necessary for survival.

How can you fully receive healing, purpose, opportunity, or happiness if your hands are full of energy-draining tasks? How can you begin a healing journey with migraines if your head is harboring bitterness, anger, or deceit? How can you thrive and be fruitful if your heart is overgrown with weeds of attachment, unforgiveness, or unresolved trauma? Just as diseased branches take away resources from the healthy plant, flourishing wellness cannot begin until the stale and detrimental stalks are examined, nurtured, or removed.

Your Pruning Plan

What area of your life feels the most draining or unfruitful? In what areas are you overcommitted or undernourished? Think in terms of unrealistic expectations, negative mindsets, physical clutter, overspending, overeating, or codependency in unhealthy relationships - whatever stands out to you the most.

How are these shriveled branches contributing to your experience with migraines?

What is blocking you from pruning this area of your life?

If you feel hesitant to prune this area, what lies beneath that feeling? What fear is preventing you from moving forward?

Pruning does not always mean eliminating a person or commitment from your life, but removing your attachment or expectation, or spending less energy, time, or resources in an area. If you were to prune this area, in what ways would your energy be revitalized, and how would your life be more fruitful or blossom?

How would a migraine-free life enhance your ability to thrive?

What relationships draw the most positive, healing energy for you? List these people or groups.

What are the qualities about this person or group that make you feel light, peaceful, or energized?

Who might you enlist to be your pruning partner? Who will keep you accountable, have your best interests in mind, and be honest with you?

In order to thrive and live a life free from migraines, you may need to remove areas, attachments, or behaviors that are sending your energy into unfruitful places. Send your valuable energy to the things that create vitality in your life. Set a date that you wish to have a healthy pruning party or at least a pruning discussion with someone you trust.

Living Your Life Purpose

What is your true calling? Do you have your good job, yet still feel empty inside? Do you feel that your life is lacking flow, purpose, or greater meaning? Do you feel stuck in a hamster wheel, but get the sense that there's something out in the world for you to accomplish? Do you ever ask yourself, "What is the point of it all?" These questions are poised inside of our innermost being to help us align our lives with our purpose for existence. Our sense of **purpose** - the substance of our being in an organized flow with clear direction - does not come from our title as a daycare provider, mom, secretary, teacher, engineer, or attorney. Instead, purpose is a deeper meaning for why we are here. You will be able to connect with and live out your authenticity by living out your life purpose.

How is life purpose relevant to migraines and other chronic diseases? Several studies have shown a strong correlation of life purpose to health outcomes. A study published by the *Journal of the American Medical Association* in 2019 showed that for people who self-reported a low sense of purpose, they were twice as likely to die prematurely than those who reported a high sense of purpose (Alimujiang et al, 2019). When people lack purpose, they may lack the motivation to practice healthy behaviors and mindsets (such as in the methods in this book). This section will help you identify, unlock, and live out your overall purpose for a fulfilling, vibrant life free of migraines.

My Journey of Purpose

When in the middle of a migraine crisis, it is hard to see purpose in the pain. Pain with purpose is somehow more acceptable, whereas pain without purpose seems to be meaningless suffering. For example, the pain of childbirth is temporary and likely results with the birth of the child. The pain of a burned finger can serve as a reminder to be more mindful while cooking. On the contrary, it is difficult to find purpose in the pain and suffering of a migraine. Many times, I would cry out and ask, "What is the point of this misery?" I can look back now and see that my suffering led to my inquiry for healing, and that inquiry led to the discovery of methods which transformed my experience with migraines. The purpose of my decades-long painful experience of suffering is to help you with yours.

It took me decades to identify my life purpose. I was not fully aware of the concept until I immersed myself into yoga teachings. As a child, I envisioned being single without children and working as a surgeon in the Air Force. I loved the idea of moving frequently to experience new cultures (the Vata in me). With my keen attention to detail and my interest in the human anatomy and physiology, a career as a surgeon seemed like the path that would bring me most satisfaction in life (the Pitta in me). However, after becoming pregnant with my daughter my senior year of high school, the trajectory of my life changed course rapidly. I was faced with new decisions on my life path, and out of haste, I decided to attend nursing school. Fast forward twenty-plus years into my professional career, I have acknowledged that my **dharma** and **ikigai** are deeper than my title, education, and experience as a nurse, firefighter, photographer, teacher, wife, mother, daughter, grandmother, and sister. After years of reflecting on what made me the happiest and feel the most fulfilled, my life purpose became crystal clear:

Empower others to achieve their greatest state of wellbeing, so that they are able to fully carry out their own mission with vitality.

The above statement, which later became my mission statement, came to me during meditation. For the first time, all my life experiences made sense. I saw common themes in my personal and professional experiences as I reflected on my life thus far. I was always the go-to person for health, wellness, and fitness advice. I have always enjoyed talking and writing. I was my happiest when I worked for myself, versus working an 8 to 5 corporate job. I found most satisfaction when I was able to lead someone to feel better and regain control of their health. I also realized that the pain I endured was something I learned from, enabling me to pass important knowledge onto others. When I put these all together, I do not just have a job title as a nurse, coach, or mother. I realize my greatest contribution is to help others to be well, so they can live out their purpose and thrive.

"The purpose of life is not to be happy. It is to be useful, to be honorable, to be compassionate, to have it make some difference that you have lived and lived well."
-Ralph Waldo Emerson

I take an unrestricted approach to understanding and living out life's purpose. Instead of neatly tucking my beliefs into a preformed box of cultural norms, I study and incorporate beliefs of different cultures and spiritual beliefs to see the common denominators. In this chapter, I will highlight principles of different cultures and spiritual paths that all lead to a similar goal: equanimity, love, peace, purpose, fulfillment, and the cessation of suffering.

The Sweet Spot of Purpose

In Buddhist philosophical teachings, a sense of purpose is referred to as **dharma**. In the Japanese culture, a deep life meaning and "sweet spot" of purpose is known as **ikigai**. Ancient yoga texts describe dharma as our true north and the role we play in the contribution to the greater good of humankind. Christians believe in the sharing of our divine spiritual gifts. Regardless of what label we give it, our purpose is rooted in our "why" for waking up each day, and the joy we find in life. We all have unique talents, personality types, and experiences that are designed to help us live out our greater purpose. Seeking a sense of purpose beyond ourselves is essential to a thriving life.

The Four Purusharthas

It is easy to get caught up in the tasks of life such as paying bills, taking the kids to school, cleaning the house, starting another diet, going to the doctor, getting the oil changed, and making time for family. In the ancient yogic texts, achieving the goal of a balanced life with high moral satisfaction is accomplished through four conditions or paths. These paths are referred to as **The Four Purusharthas**, which are the four aims or desires of the soul. *Purusha* in Sanskrit is translated as "the soul, original source of the universe", and *artha* means "aim, cause, motion, the purpose of, or ability". It is suggested that, when these four paths are aligned, we are better able to handle stress in life while simultaneously feeling a greater sense of purpose.

When we are living out our dharma, we feel fulfilled, energized, focused, and in our "flow."

The first of these paths is **dharma**, which is composed of our life purpose, ethics, morals, and our duty to contribute to the world around us. Dharma gives us our sense of truth and responsibility to "do good" in the world. The root of the word *dharma* means to "firm, establish, or create structure" (Dowdle, 2010). Throughout our lives we may have many dharmas, depending on our roles at the time. If you are a parent, it may be part of your dharma to raise a responsible and respectful child, so that they can live out their dharma. If you are in a position or role that you dread, or the role is affecting your health in negative ways, this could mean that it is not in alignment with your dharma. When dharma is out of balance, we may feel frustrated, stuck, bored, depressed, or resentful. When we are living out our dharma, we feel fulfilled, energized, focused, and in our "flow."

Kama is the second path that can lead us to a place of moral satisfaction in life. Like the principles of ikigai, kama is best described as our desire or pleasure. When kama and dharma align, we can find fulfillment, joy, and pleasure in our purpose. Although dharma may involve a degree of sacrifice, kama makes the sacrifice worthy and enjoyable. If your dharma is to provide a safe, loving, stable environment for your children, we can practice kama while we do the dishes. Instead of saying "I have to do the dishes", we can flip the script and align our dharma with kama by saying "I am able to provide a clean home for my children, and dirty dishes mean nourished bodies." Practicing kama in daily tasks may take time, as it takes practice to stay present, mindful, and gracious in the seemingly mundane.

Artha is the third of the four aims of purpose. Representing secure economic and material comfort, artha can easily become unbalanced in a society of greed, selfishness, or the constant seeking of success or material gain. One who is on a path of freedom from material attachments understands that artha is not excess, but a comfortable means to live a balanced life. Artha is not just money and material possessions; instead, it is the foundation to have enough resources to care for yourself and family and to execute your purpose. Artha represents the relationships, environment, assets, love, health, and knowledge necessary to live a purpose-filled life. When we do work that we love while filling a greater need outside of ourselves, we are making the conscious decision to align our energy with our divine purpose. It is then that artha will flow.

The last of *The Four Purusharthas* is **moksha**. When we fulfill our dharma (purpose) with the support of kama (passion, pleasure) and artha (resources), we can achieve moksha. This pinnacle of fulfilled purpose is our true essence and freedom from being stuck in a cycle of emotional or physical pain. Often, we get stuck in self-limiting beliefs that we were "born this way," and "nothing will ever change." Some find comfort in staying stuck in an unchanged story, because change seems too challenging. Moksha also represents freedom from the grip of suffering.

Positive thoughts become positive beliefs, and those positive beliefs become positive behaviors.

As we work towards removing toxic influences, aligning the systems of our body-mind, and dialing in our purpose, we can reach a transformational state that is free from suffering. **Suffering** is a passing experience. We do not have to stay in the state of suffering. At some point, when we are sick and tired of being sick and tired, we can make the conscious choice to identify, break free, and remold the suffering cycle into a life that is free from migraines. For some, this process requires deep work to work through traumas and pain. As you take one step in front of the other in the direction of breaking free from migraines, be patient, kind, and loving with yourself on your journey.

Ikigai

The Japanese city of Okinawa is one of a handful of regions around the world known as the Blue Zones, where most people live past 100 years old in relatively superior health. In Okinawa, an above average life expectancy is tied to **ikigai**, which is one of nine health practices for longevity identified by Dan Buettner in his book, *The Blue Zones* (2012). Studies show that having a clear ikigai helps close the gap on poor health outcomes, as those with a clear ikigai have less psychosocial issues such as depression and anxiety, and experience improved sleep quality. Since we know there is a relationship between emotional, mental, and neurological health with migraines, aligning our daily life practices with our ikigai could help reduce the burden of the disease.

FINDING YOUR IKIGAI

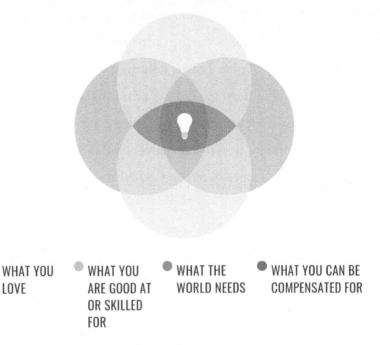

| 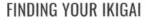 WHAT YOU LOVE | WHAT YOU ARE GOOD AT OR SKILLED FOR | WHAT THE WORLD NEEDS | WHAT YOU CAN BE COMPENSATED FOR |

Our values, beliefs, talents, and personality drive our ikigai. Ikigai can be described as a clear sense of purpose that is aligned with what you are good at, what you enjoy, what the world needs, and what you can be compensated for. The visual of the sweet spot of ikigai can help you identify these core areas to unlock your purpose and enhance your quality of life.

Suffering and the Four Noble Truths

Migraineurs have experienced suffering of the mind, body, and spirit. Regardless of the type or duration, migraines can leave a person feeling completely defeated. What is the purpose of suffering? Based on Buddhist philosophy*, the **Four Noble Truths** help to give a sense of direction and purpose to pain and suffering. Gautama Buddha was an ordinary person who lived in India 2,600 years ago; he became a philosopher, meditation teacher, and spiritual guide. He later developed the teachings of these core principles, universally known as the *Four Noble Truths.*

For many people, Buddhism is not a religion, but a way of living for a peaceful, generous, and enjoyable life.

These four truths all relate to aspects of suffering. The first of these is *Dukkha*, which speaks on the truth or **reason for suffering**. While it is common to understand suffering related to emotional or physical pain, which migraines are an example of, suffering in this context can further be defined as "insatiable needs, stress, or loss." We established earlier that pain is an inevitable part of life. However, our response to the pain defines our perception of the pain experience. Dukkha affirms that, although pain is experienced, it is temporary. When we identify ourselves with our pain, we are essentially making our pain permanent. When we look outward for an ease of suffering (going to doctors, taking medications, blaming others, abusing drugs or alcohol, etc.), we ignore our internal power and our role in the suffering.

The second Noble Truth is *Samudāya*, which is the **cause of suffering** rooted in attachment, desire, or ego. This is a tough one - not everyone is ready to conceptualize the possibility that their expectations could be causing their suffering. A person who experiences migraines may suffer because they expect to be able to live each day pain-free, but when that expectation is not met, they suffer. You may say the more logical explanation is that suffering exists purely as a result of the physical sensations occurring in the body during a migraine. This explanation certainly holds truth, otherwise most of the content in this book would be unnecessary. The Buddhist way of thinking simply asserts that suffering can also come about due to ideas or ideals being threatened and lost. Both physical and mental sensations come into play when we enter a state of suffering. It is unthinkable to separate the two.

The Buddha believed there were three causes of suffering: 1) greed, attachment, or unreasonable desire; 2) unawareness or misunderstanding of the true nature of life; and 3) destructive, impulsive behaviors. I have personally experienced the suffering these can bring; the cause of my prolonged suffering for years was related to *what I thought my life should be.* I was attempting to separate my physical pain from my emotional state, which manifested as unforgiveness, negative mindsets, bitterness, and perfectionism. My daily mantra would reverberate, "Why ME?"

Now that I am on the path to connecting my emotions, mind, body, and spirit as one, I appreciate that suffering is temporal. I understand that my pain is an experience for me through which to learn, grow, slow down, or help others, to lead to my purpose. Although the pain we experience

324 | *The Migraine Method*

can feel overwhelming, it is transient. What we have inside of us is greater and more potent than temporary pain.

After one can identify the root cause of their suffering, they will be able to find ways of ending that suffering. The third Noble Truth, called *Nirodha*, points toward this end of suffering. According to the Buddha, the way to ease suffering is to let go from unhealthy attachments that blind us from seeing our truth. We can live a life free from migraines when we break away from the attachment of suffering. This may seem paradoxical. For some, even though not easily admitted, there is an odd comfort in being unwell by attaching the illness or disease to our identity, claiming, "it's just who I am." I recall simultaneously hating migraines yet savoring the comfort I gained while being unwell; instead of seeking healing from within myself, I convinced myself that I was trapped in a chronicle of suffering and relied on external soothing.

Living a life free from migraines does not mean that we will never again experience a migraine. Rather, living free from migraines means releasing all attachments and separating our existence from the migraine. It means that we have the power within ourselves to act rather than letting the attacks overcome us. It means we can observe our bodily responses, equipped with the knowledge and mental strength to build resilience. It means being able to apply tried-and-tested methods when the time of need arises. It means taking ownership of how we speak to ourselves and what we believe about ourselves. When we detach from negative mindsets, unhealthy behaviors, toxic environments, and draining relationships; when we take everything holding us back and replace it with practices that nourish our mind, body, and spirit; the state we will then find ourselves in is a thriving existence free from suffering.

The last of the Noble Truths is *Magga*, a path to enlightenment and freedom from suffering. Magga promotes living a balanced life where we avoid excess or depravity. In this state of contentment, a person can live a life free of suffering and without judgement, so that their responses to life's experiences come from a place of love, compassion, and acceptance. The **Eightfold Path** is designed to lead one to the end of suffering, while living a balanced life. One might even see similarities of this path to the Ten Commandments in the Bible. Regardless of the title or origin of the steps of the path, aligning yourself with these principles will support you on your path to freedom from migraines. This path is not chronological; instead, each of these steps support the other steps. The approaches of *The Migraine Method* are mirrored from the Eightfold Path; in order to reach a state of freedom from migraines, these mindsets and methods should be incorporated into your everyday life. The Buddha taught each step of this path in a way that can be compared to shoes we wear throughout life. Once we outgrow a pair of shoes, we no longer need that pair. We move on to wearing shoes that fit our current state of growth.

The Eightfold Path to Enlightenment to End Suffering from Migraines

Right Understanding or View

One of the most difficult realities to accept is that the world is not all that we perceive it to be. With a right outlook, we seek to understand the world, the meaning of life, and our purpose as it is - not as we wish or desire it to be. Perhaps this step necessitates us to look inward and uncover the root of our disease. Maybe it is looking within and being intentional to calm the brain, instead of seeking the rescue of another doctor, another medication, or another quick fix. Having the right understanding is seeking to understand our role in the migraine experience, but also our role in the universe.

In order to work towards a life without suffering, every time the symptoms of a migraine are experienced, we must shift our inquisition from "Why is this happening to me?" to "What am I supposed to learn from this experience?" This was probably the hardest shift for me while working towards freedom from migraines. Every now and then I still struggle in this area, especially when it comes to the upright versus corrupt in the world. I feel that since I have a noble heart and lead with moral intent, everyone else in the world must also, and at times I become discouraged when I hear of the corruption or merciless behaviors of others. I also struggle with unplanned surprises. Growing up, I felt like my world was unpredictable and unstable, so I feel secure when my environment is predictable and steady. Now, I recognize that suffering occurs when my attachment to my expectations rattles my core values.

What is your definition of suffering? What belief or understanding of the world do you have? In what ways is it a limiting belief? How do your beliefs about your migraine experience shape your life? In what ways do you prioritize daily steps toward inner healing? It breaks my heart when I hear migraineurs say, "I am glad it worked for you, it won't work for me." Or "I tried meditation and yoga; it didn't work for me. I just have to get on a higher dose of medication instead." When we have suffered so much for so long, I know it is hard to believe that some degree of improvement is possible. But I challenge you to consider, in an empathetic and compassionate way, what role does your response play in suffering? When we unfold the truth of the meaning of life and choose to not limit ourselves in the suffering of our present condition, we can expand our awareness and shift our perspective at any given time.

Right Intention

Taking a deeper look into our commitment and motive is the second path to freedom from suffering. Having the right intent must come from the heart, and it must be of pure inclination. For example: my compelling intention to write this book and share my experiences and research with others was not for fame or notoriety, but to help others on their path to whole wellness and freedom from suffering. Right intent takes dedication, passion, commitment, and persistence. In order to free yourself from migraines, you must be ready, committed, and have a passion for letting go of toxic lifestyle thoughts, beliefs, choices, and patterns.

Right Speech

As I have reiterated in previous chapters, our cells are listening to our thoughts. Everything in and around us is energy; it responds according to the information it receives. Having the right speech with the right intent builds the groundwork for freedom from suffering. Whether it is your verbal speech or your mental monologue, speaking positivity and encouragement to self and others is essential to aligning your mind and body into wellness. As Jesus spoke, "Out of the abundance of the heart the mouth speaks" (Matthew 12:34). Motivation for all that we say, do, or think comes from heart (intent). Could you agree that it is by divine design that the mouth is nestled between the heart and the head?

Right Action

Once you have aligned your vision, intent, and speech towards freedom from suffering, the next step is action. This step is our propelling moral compass and requires due diligence to do no harm to self or others. Reading this book and opening your mind to pursuing healing from within may be a huge shift of thought for you. Wherever you are on your path is right where you need to be. Perhaps your next step is to move forward with action steps and commit to your health by incorporating the steps contained herein. Which method are you excited to start? Which step are you putting off because it seems too difficult? When your actions are rooted in the first three steps of the Eightfold Path, your life begins to take shape to end suffering.

Right Livelihood

This next step embraces a sound mind in a sound body. The path to freedom from suffering is not just a physical or emotional journey, but a spiritual path as well. When you have identified and aligned your values, purpose, understanding, heart, speech, and action steps together, you are living your dharma. According to the Buddha, your life and your work should not create harm to you or others. Remember, too, that your work and your dharma are beyond a typical employment. Your work is your contribution to the world, which can take many different forms.

For example, my brother is a lively 23-year-old man living with high-functioning autism. Through the lens of disability, some may say that his contributions are minimal, since he does not hold typical employment. However, he is a part-time college student, helps our mother with household chores, and is a self-made comedian. His contribution is helping our single mother with yardwork and housework and eliciting laughter to those around him through his jokes and storytelling. When I ask him about his contentment in life, he tells me consistently, "I am living my best life every day." Perhaps restricted mindsets are a more widespread infirmity than a disability.

Right Effort

The right effort is the oomph, gumption, and bravery behind what you do. I wasn't a cheerleader growing up, but I would imagine that a cheerleader with enthusiasm, excitement, passion, and fervor can get the crowd motivated better than a pessimistic one. I came a similar situation while at the store recently. Although I could not see this woman, I clearly heard her stocking the shelves saying, "This is so ****ing stupid. Who would do this work? Ugh, I can't wait to get out of here." She continued with her lamentation; but I did not stick around for much of it. What I did hear, though, was a clear example of someone channeling their available energy into an unconstructive outcome. How could she enjoy her day if that is how she described it?

We all have days that are worse than others. I am sure you have been able to relate to the woman at the store at least a few times throughout your life. We can have mini tantrums, but then we must move on if we expect a different outcome. Choosing a path without suffering is living a life with balanced effort and enthusiasm - using our energy for positive outcomes, not negative ones. Just like the story about Goldilocks and the Three Bears, right in the middle seems to be the most effective long-term. Not too hot, not too cold. Our attitude and outlook steer the trajectory of our day.

Right Mindfulness

In chapter eight I shared at length the importance of mindfulness and meditation for migraines. According to the principles of the Eightfold Path, mindfulness helps us to stay present and not skip ahead or dwell on the past. Anxiety is stress or fear of the future, while depression is stress or regret about the past; mindfulness helps us to evade both. Mindfulness is not blocking out painful experiences, but instead, being present and returning our focus to things we can see, hear, or feel. When we are present, we can identify and capture the thoughts, beliefs, and behaviors that have gotten us to this very moment. As humans, our basic need of survival means that the brain, body, and mind will do whatever it takes to survive, even if those actions are unhealthy or destructive. By adopting healthy coping skills such as mindfulness, we can live in the present moment, which is the only moment that truly exists. Where is yesterday? Where is tomorrow? Right *now* is the only moment that we have.

Right concentration

A mind free from clutter can focus on what needs to be achieved. When we have not cleared the space to receive, it becomes more cluttered and chaotic. However, when we remove the barriers, excuses, hindrances, and self-limiting beliefs, we can open ourselves to receive wisdom and loving kindness to move closer to the end of suffering. These principles of mindfulness and concentration help us to see the world and our experiences for how they really are, not how we have been inclined to see them. What we focus on becomes our center; and our body systems follows our concentration. If the mind is distressed and exhausted, the body will mirror the mind. The more we focus on the disease, the more intense it becomes.

You have the power to refocus your lens to experience joy in life. I know firsthand that it is challenging to find joy in the middle of a migraine. Joy is internal; happiness is based on external events. Joy is immovable; happiness can be conditional. The purpose in your experience of pain and suffering is for you to discover joy and peace. As you move through your path to the end of suffering, be present, be loving, be kind, and be patient with *you*.

Identify, Align, and Live Your Purpose

Use these questions to reflect on your purpose:

- Those who meet the morning with resistance may be misaligned with their purpose. Those who wake up with energy and excitement are better positioned to make an impact on the world around them. When you first wake up, what is your mood?

- Do you believe that purpose is a destiny we are born with, a choice, or a combination of the two? Why?

- Make a list of at least three of your natural talents that you enjoy using. For example: great at growing plants, able to refurbish furniture, exceptional at speaking to large audiences, photographing nature, selling clothing, building and constructing, or writing. Think back to your childhood and look for themes.

  I am good at and enjoy:

  1. _____
  2. _____
  3. _____

- Make a list of at least three times in your life when you felt the happiest. Be specific. Think about experiences where time seemed to stand still and you felt fulfilled, joyful, and content. This serves the purposes of *kama and dharma.*

  1. _____
  2. _____
  3. _____

- Make a list of at least three causes, people, or groups you are passionate about. For example, are you passionate about reducing environmental waste, or is it important to you to advocate for children that are abused?

1. _____

2. _____

3. _____

- What do you believe is your role in contributing value to your family, community, society, or the world?

- What is the legacy that you wish to leave behind? What do you want to be remembered for by the people who know you?

- What is something that the world needs, that aligns with your values, beliefs, passions, and talents? For example, the world may need someone who enjoys writing and telling stories to bring joy and laughter in the form of jokes or short stories.

  A person who is good at painting and passionate about helping others may offer their skill to bring joy through artwork.

- What is a gap that you could fill, that is aligned with your talents, values, beliefs, and the needs of the world, that you could be compensated for? *Compensation is more than money - it can also be an exchange of energy or gratitude. This exchange serves the purpose of artha.*

- Write out your life purpose statement by filling in the blanks.

I feel most alive when I am:

_____

The thing that gets me excited to wake up in the morning is being able to:

_____

I desire to leave a legacy and my impact on the world by:

_____

Right now, I am choosing to let go of the toxic, self-limiting belief that:

_____

.

Conclusion

A summary of the essential points to take with you
on your wellness journey.

The Purpose and Practice of The Migraine Method

I HOPE YOU HAVE FOUND VALUABLE PRINCIPLES worth taking to the drawing board to implement into your life. My hope is that the lessons I have learned after 24 years of suffering and searching for my purpose will bring you to a place of inquisition, a place from which you can begin taking steps toward the end of suffering. Remember, this book is not a cure-all. Be patient with yourself as you navigate untapped parts of yourself. Only through consistency, perseverance, and hope will you end suffering to live a thriving life free of migraines. These methods do not have a pinnacle of achievement, but instead will grant you access to a more vibrant, flourishing life.

In my early 20s I thought I would hit 35 and "arrive." I was disappointed when at 37, I was still making mistakes and learning new things about myself. I found that there are layers to the self that are sometimes only expressed under fire. I would never have been able to write this book had I not suffered for the last two decades. I had to become thirsty and hungry enough for a different way of living before I could seek and find the truth in healing.

There may be parts of this book that are not for you. Perhaps there are some concepts that you had not considered as an influential factor in your migraine experience. Approach all of it with an open mind, knowing that you have nothing to lose by implementing strategies to better yourself. If it helps, don't make getting rid of your migraines the main goal; strive for a healthy mind and body, and your migraine experience will improve naturally from there. I hope you will return to this book often and use it as a guide for a thriving life. I believe the principles in these pages will evoke a desire in you to seek more truth, starting you on a journey you won't want to end. Be slightly obsessed with the truth that a life without migraines is possible.

The Take-Home

Before you close the cover and head into your personal wellness journey, I will briefly summarize the past 300-odd pages into their take-home points. We have covered a lot! Let's break it down a bit:

Wellness is the barometer of the mind-body. Migraines are a warning sign that our wellness is out of balance. The physiological, psychological, and spiritual framework of homeostasis allows us to quantify wellness in terms of resilience, which is the ability to adapt continuously to internal and external situations. Health may be a state of being that is free of disease or disorder, but wellness is living a thriving life with optimal health. A person can be in near perfect health, but not be well. A person can have a disease or disorder but feel well when they are living harmoniously. In order to maintain a positive balance of health and wellness for a thriving life free of migraines, the wear and tear on our nervous system must not exceed our capability of adapting to stress, whether the stress is in the past or in the present.

Less impact of chronic disease equals an increase in quality of life.

Our fiercest struggles while suffering from migraines will ultimately lead us to our victories, relief, and purpose. Within this context, **the onset of disease or disorder (such as migraines) starts when the brain, mind, or body's adaptive processes deteriorate.** Often, we do not even realize how badly beat up our systems are until illnesses surface. In retrospect, we can piece together the unresolved trauma, repetitive stress, toxic emotions, unhealthy relationships, inflammatory foods, lack of quality sleep, or genetics that powerfully influenced the breakdown of our body and mind. As we learn to understand the brain and what systems are in place to keep us safe and alive, we can begin to see that our conditioned stress responses were for our survival. Resilience is a springboard for a migraine-free life. Our chosen lifestyle plays an important role in maintaining a strong capacity for resilience.

Remember that **your story is your story.** You have a uniquely fashioned lens through which to view your world, including the pain you experience and how you experience it. The way you react to stress is influenced by your experiences, your core values, and your biology. If your stress response patterns are causing you to be unwell, you can make a change and pry yourself from those unhealthy patterns. You have learned about how the brain responds to stress or threats in the mind or body for survival with a surge of chemicals, electrical impulses, inflammation, and blood vessel changes. You are now fully equipped to start recalibrating and retraining the brain for harmonious resilience.

Resilience is the springboard for a migraine-free life.

One of the most essential practices to a migraine-free life is a truly restful sleep. As told in the Bible, Jesus took naps to restore physical, emotional, mental, and spiritual well-being. It is time to give yourself a calming sleep space, an essential prerequisite to restoring the brain's energy, rejuvenating tissues, and rebalancing hormones. As you establish a nightly routine and sleep kit to prime and condition yourself for sleep, you will be able to help build optimal resilience to stress.

Stress is ubiquitous in the world we live in. Thankfully, **you do not have to absorb and respond to every stressor as an unrivaled threat.** The brain's job is to act as a security guard or surveillance camera, constantly monitoring the environment in which we live. As you build resilience and balance your internal systems, stressors do not have a space to build up. You will be able to capture out of control thoughts that present as worries, fears, resentment, anger, jealousy, or unforgiveness. Although you may not be able to control external stressors such as unpredictable changes or major life events, **the more you use interoception to monitor how stress** affects your mind and body, the more in-tune you will become to what keeps you well.

Without much prompting, you could probably write down the three types of foods that make you feel bloated, heavy, weighed down, or in pain. You don't need an honorary medical degree in nutrition to know there is a reason you feel unwell after eating certain foods. **Listen to your body.** Now that you are armed with the tools to remove migraine triggering foods, decide for your own sake to act on what you have learned. Before long, you can inoculate the gut with beneficial bacteria, repair inflammation in the gut, reduce cravings, and rebalance the immune and hormone system with the foods that give you optimum energy and sustenance.

At any given moment of your day, hormones are rising and falling without your awareness. Fortunately, humans do not have to think about or self-monitor thyroid hormones, reproductive hormones, appetite hormones, or mood-altering hormones. Can you imagine if you had to monitor every cellular transaction in your body? We would be a complete mess. Hormone balance is so delicate and yet crucial to quality of life. Still, there are ways we can aid our hormonal balance in how we live and the way we treat our bodies. **From self-talk to serotonin, hormones govern the operative expression of health in the body.**

Many of the body's processes are automatic, but the breath is the one process that you can simultaneously control or allow to happen naturally. The breath responds accordingly whether you are stressed or calm. **How you breathe is how you live.** The ancient sages of yogic teachings believed that if you can control your breath, you can control your responses to the changes of life. Developing a mindful movement practice such as yoga, meditation, or simply controlled breathing will help you build stress buoyancy to subdue migraines.

Stress alters DNA. How you respond to stress, what foods you eat, how you live, and what you allow in your life either turns on or turns off genes. Cellular stress in the form of oxidation can create an inflammatory platform for migraines. Aging starts at the cellular level, and you have power over how your cells age. Reducing chemical exposures, eating clean foods, and choosing supplements that minimize inflammation and oxidative stress in the body will help to change your epigenetic signature and reduce the risk of migraines.

Just as your DNA has a distinctive "signature," what do you want your mark on the world to be? What do you want to be known for? How do your relationships influence your levels of perceived stress? What is your greater purpose in this life? My hope is that these questions have sparked a curiosity in you to dig deeper and **take inventory of how your values, relationships, and purpose have influenced your experience with migraines.** The million-dollar question is, who are you without migraines?

Collectively, **mind-body practices are the first line of care for all parts of the self**. Ayurvedic practices can be viewed as the way one lives a steady, balanced, nurturing life, with a more wholesome state of being as the natural self. When we care for and nourish ourselves through daily routines that rejuvenate the body-mind, we can feel more grounded, balanced, and whole. As we find our individual rhythm and honor our body-mind instead of allowing toxic practices, substances, thoughts, people, and circumstances in our life, we create the potential for positive change towards a migraine-free life. Ayurveda gives the space to calm the nervous system before the day begins and sets the direction of the cells to fire and wire together in an advantageous pattern.

Finally, consider the metaphor of the weed and its roots. There is little benefit in snapping a weed off by the stem or simply trimming its leaves. We must **pull the roots** and cut the weed off from its source; likewise, we must treat the cause of suffering rather than continually suppressing our symptoms. Ending suffering is not for our benefit, but instead for us to contribute our purpose for the good of mankind. Just as a flower blossoms and shares an aroma for others to enjoy, **allow the harmony of your mind, body, and spirit to be your fragrance.** Live by this principle and see your migraine-free life blossom.

May you be safe,
may you live with joy and ease,
may you live one hundred years,
and may you be free from suffering.

SECTION FOUR

Additional Resources

Yoga Poses for Doshas

In English and Sanskrit

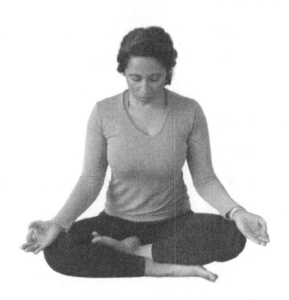

Easy Pose *(Sukhasana)*

Vata, Pitta, Kapha

Use caution with sciatica.

Avoid this pose with knee arthritis or knee surgery.

May use a cushion or blanket to elevate the hips. Practice with eyes open if during a severe migraine or anxiety.

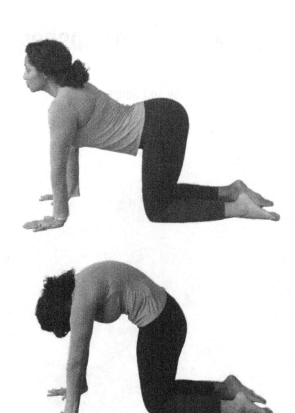

Cat / Cow *(Marjaiasana / Bitilasana)*

Vata, Pitta

Use with caution and move slowly during a migraine.

Do not hold the breath.

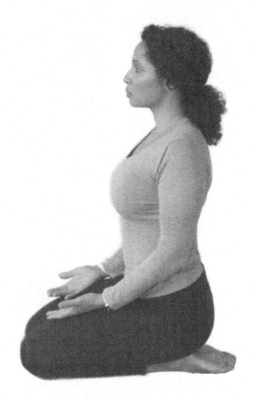

Thunderbolt Pose *(Vajrasana)*

Vata

Elevate hips with a blanket if there is ankle or knee discomfort.

Avoid if you have severe arthritic knees.

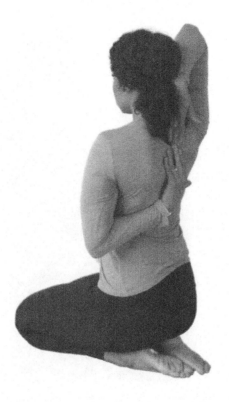

Cow Face Arms *(Gomukhasana)*

Kapha

Take it slow if there is any shoulder stiffness. The hands do not have to touch. Avoid this pose in severe shoulder injury.

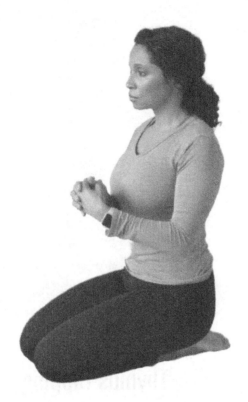

Wrist and Ankle Warm-ups

Vata

Softly rotate the wrists and ankles in a circular motion.

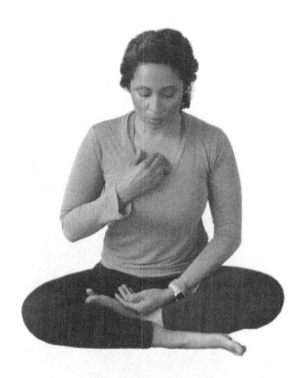

Thymus Tapping

Kapha

Gently tap the center of the breastbone with the fingertips for 15-20 seconds. Use caution with active conditions of the immune system.

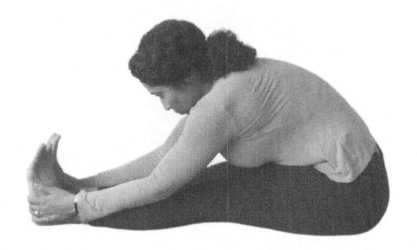

Seated Forward Bend *(Paschimottanasana)*

Pitta

Avoid this pose with an active slipped disc, hernias, or pregnancy.

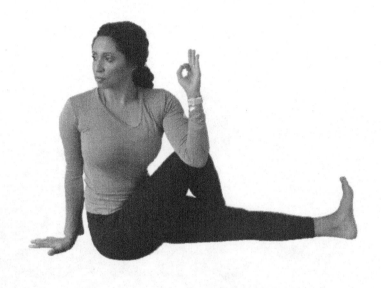

Sage Marichi III *(Marichyasana III)*

Pitta, Kapha

Avoid twisting with spinal injuries or pregnancy.

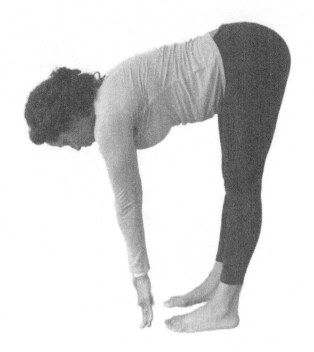

Half Forward Bend *(Ardha Uttanasana)*

Pitta, Kapha

Use caution with hamstring or lower back injuries or hernias.

Fold from the hips not the lower back.

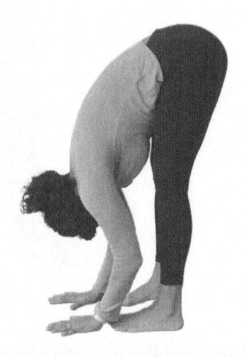

Forward Bend *(Uttanasana)*

Pitta

Use caution with hamstring, knee, or lower back injuries. Fold from the hips, not the lower back. Avoid during an active migraine.

Avoid immediately after a meal.

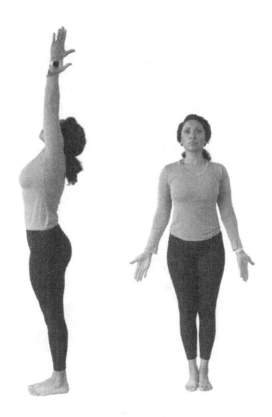

Extended Mountain Pose & Mountain Pose

(Utthita Tadasana & Tadasana)

Vata, Pitta

Do not lock knees out, keep a soft micro bend in the knees. Stack the head over the heart, heart over the hips. Softly grip the floor with the entire sole of the foot. Maintain a soft gaze.

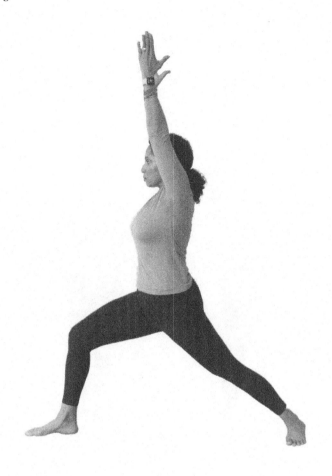

Warrior I *(Virabhadrasana I)*

Vata, Pitta, Kapha

Use caution with knee or hip injuries. Maintain breath awareness and do not hold the breath.

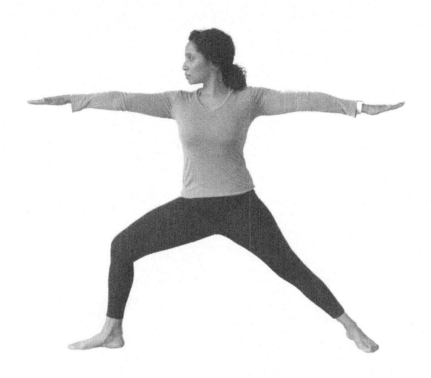

Warrior II *(Virabhadrasana II)*

Pitta, Kapha

Use caution with hip injuries or weakness. Do not hold this pose for long with heart conditions.

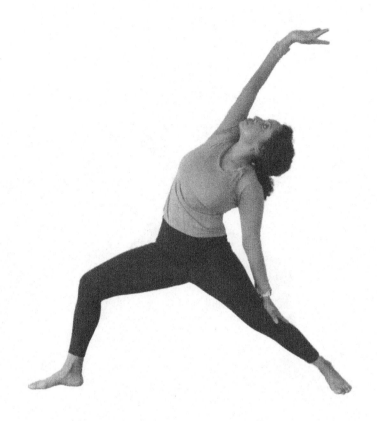

Reverse Warrior *(Viparita Virabhadrasana)*

Pitta, Kapha

Avoid this pose with spinal conditions, severe vertigo, or heart conditions.

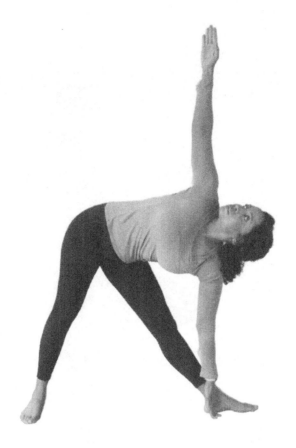

Triangle Pose *(Trikonasana)*

Vata, Pitta, Kapha

*Use caution with spine conditions, joint mobility conditions, beyond 2nd
trimester pregnancy, blood pressure issues, or heart conditions. May use a block
on the floor for the bottom hand.*

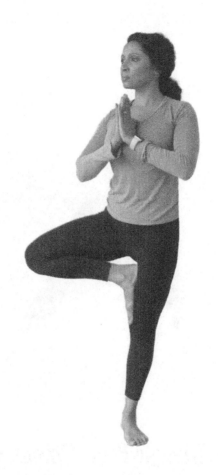

Tree Pose *(Vrksasana)*

Pitta, Kapha

Use caution as this will challenge balance, may use a wall for support.

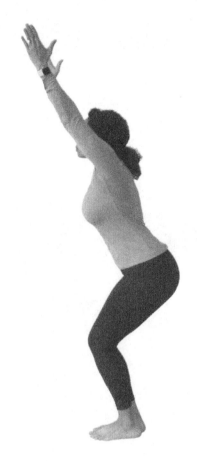

Chair Pose *(Utkatasana)*

Vata, Pitta, Kapha

Use caution with acute knee injuries or an active headache.

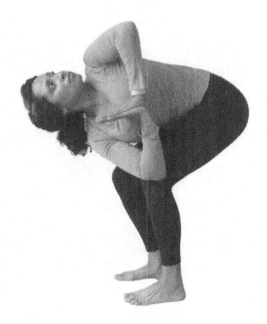

Revolved Chair Pose *(Parivrtta Utkatasana)*

Pitta, Kapha

Avoid twisting during pregnancy or with severe heart conditions.

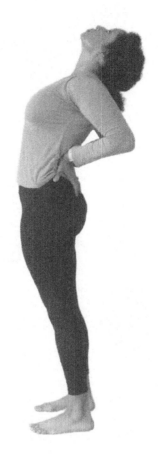

Standing Backbend Pose *(Anuvittasana)*

Vata, Pitta

Avoid deep backbends with severe vertigo,

high blood pressure, or neck injuries.

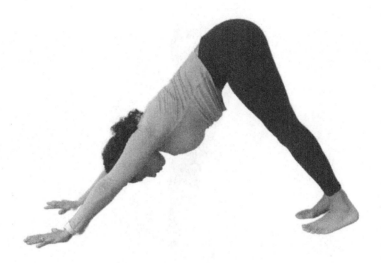

Downward Facing Dog
(Adho Mukha Svanasana)

Vata, Pitta

Use caution with high blood pressure, heart disease, or vertigo.

Come out of this pose slowly to allow the blood to flow easily.

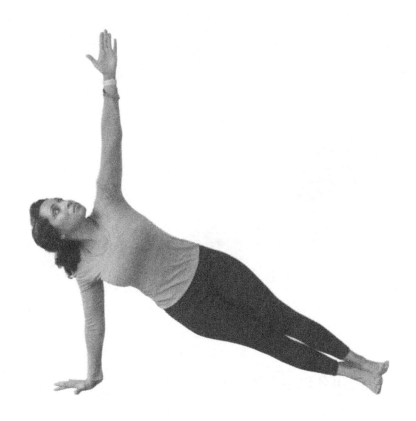

Side Plank Pose *(Vasisthasana)*

Pitta

May use a block for support or come down to forearm for wrist conditions or pregnancy. Use the wall for support. Avoid this pose with recent abdominal surgery, herniated discs, or carpal tunnel.

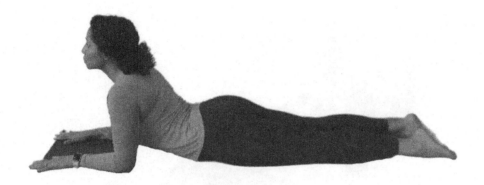

Cobra on Forearms Pose *(Bhujangasana)*

Vata, Pitta, Kapha

Do not practice during pregnancy or within 3-6 months postpartum.

Avoid if you suffer from any injury to the shoulder, neck, or spine.

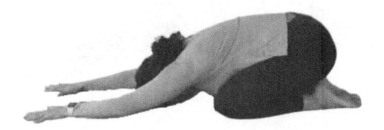

Child Pose *(Balasana)*

Pitta, Kapha

Avoid during pregnancy, knee injuries, stomach issues, or ankle injuries.

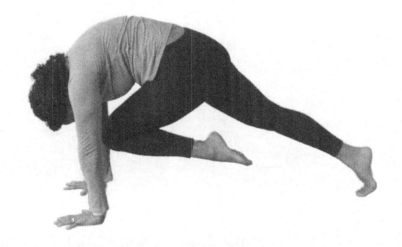

Knee to Nose Pose *(Phalakasana Variation)*

Pitta

Use caution with injuries of the shoulder, knee, wrist, abdomen, or spine.

Avoid during an active migraine, vertigo, or blood pressure issues.

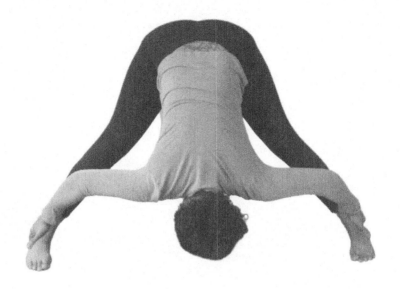

Wide Leg Forward Bend

(Prasarita Padottanasana)

Pitta, Kapha

Avoid this pose with injuries of the head, shoulder, neck, hips, or knees.
Avoid during the surgical recovery period. Use caution during active migraine
or with blood pressure conditions.

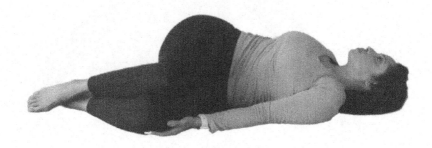

Supine Spinal Twist Pose II

(Supta Matsyendrasana II)

Vata, Pitta

Use caution with slipped discs, or injury to the neck, head, shoulders, back, hips, or knees. Use pillows for support between the knees or under the head.

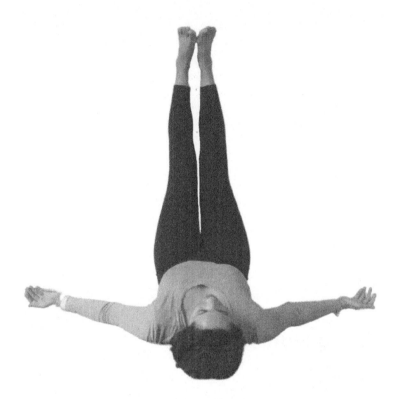

Legs Up the Wall Pose *(Viparita Karani)*

Vata, Pitta

Avoid beyond the 2nd trimester of pregnancy.

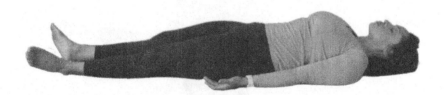

Corpse Pose *(Savasana)*

Vata, Pitta, Kapha

Avoid beyond the 2nd trimester of pregnancy. May recline side-lying with pillow in between knees, or on back with pillow under knees to support the lower back.

Resources

Resources are provided for informational purposes only. This list is not exhaustive and does not serve as endorsement or of any companies, websites, products, or sources.

Ayurveda

Banyan Botanicals

Products to support an ayurvedic lifestyle.

Website: https://www.banyanbotanicals.com

Telephone: 1-800-953-6424

Email: info@banyanbotanicals.com

Health Coaching and Corporate Wellness

Elizabeth Priller Consulting

Website: https://www.elizabethpriller.com

Connect on Facebook, Instagram, LinkedIn, and YouTube

Courses

The Mind-Body Resilience Institute

https://elizabeth-priller-consulting.teachable.com

Migraine Meditations

www.elizabethpriller.com/migrainemeditation

Migraine Relief and Supplements

The Zōk Relief Device

https://zokrelief.com

NOW Foods

Website: https://www.nowfoods.com

Corporate Offices

244 Knollwood Drive Bloomingdale, IL 60108

Telephone: 1-888-669-3663

Life Extension

Website: https://www.lifeextension.com

Telephone: 1-800-678-8989

Sleep Apps

SleepyTime

https://sleepyti.me

Sleep Cycle Alarm Clock

https://www.sleepcycle.com

References

Aggarwal, M., Puri, V., & Puri, S. (2012). Serotonin and CGRP in migraine. *Annals of Neurosciences, 19*(2), 88–94. https://doi.org/10.5214/ans.0972.7531.12190210

Al-Quliti, K. W., & Assaedi, E. S. (2016). New advances in prevention of migraine. Review of current practice and recent advances. *Neurosciences (Riyadh, Saudi Arabia), 21*(3), 207–214. https://doi.org/10.17712/nsj.2016.3.20150506

Alegría-Torres, J. A., Baccarelli, A., & Bollati, V. (2011). Epigenetics and lifestyle. *Epigenomics, 3*(3), 267–277. https://doi.org/10.2217/epi.11.22

Alimujiang, A., Wiensch, A., Boss, J., Fleischer, N. L., Mondul, A. M., Mclean, K., . . . Pearce, C. L. (2019). Association Between Life Purpose and Mortality Among US Adults Older Than 50 Years. *JAMA Network Open, 2*(5). doi:10.1001/jamanetworkopen.2019.4270

Alshak, M. (2019, May 13). Neuroanatomy, Sympathetic Nervous System. Retrieved June 22, 2020, from https://www.ncbi.nlm.nih.gov/books/NBK542195/

Anda, R., Tietjen, G., Schulman, E., Felitti, V., & Croft, J. (2010). Adverse childhood experiences and frequent headaches in adults. *Headache, 50*(9), 1473–1481. https://doi.org/10.1111/j.1526-4610.2010.01756.x

Arzani, M., Jahromi, S. R., Ghorbani, Z., Vahabizad, F., Martelletti, P., Ghaemi, A., Sacco, S., Togha, M., & School of Advanced Studies of the European Headache Federation (EHF-SAS) (2020). Gut-brain Axis and migraine headache: a comprehensive review. *The Journal of Headache and Pain, 21*(1), 15. https://doi.org/10.1186/s10194-020-1078-9

Avnon, Y. (2004). Autonomic asymmetry in migraine: Augmented parasympathetic activation in left unilateral migraineurs. *Brain, 127*(9), 2099-2108. doi:10.1093/brain/awh236

Bayles, B., Usatine, R. (2009, December 15). Evening Primrose Oil. Retrieved June 22, 2020, from https://www.aafp.org/afp/2009/1215/p1405.html

Benedict, C., Vogel, H., Jonas, W., Woting, A., Blaut, M., Schürmann, A., & Cedernaes, J. (2016). Gut microbiota and glucometabolic alterations in response to recurrent partial sleep deprivation in normal-weight young individuals. *Molecular Metabolism, 5*(12), 1175–1186. https://doi.org/10.1016/j.molmet.2016.10.003

Blackburn, E. H., & Epel, E. S. (2012). Too toxic to ignore. *Nature, 490*(7419), 169-171. doi:10.1038/490169a

Bond, D. S., Roth, J., Nash, J. M., & Wing, R. R. (2011). Migraine and obesity: epidemiology, possible mechanisms and the potential role of weight loss treatment. *Obesity Reviews: An Official Journal Of The International Association for the Study of Obesity, 12*(5), e362–e371. https://doi.org/10.1111/j.1467-789X.2010.00791.x

Buettner, D. (2012). *The Blue Zones: 9 lessons for living longer from the people who've lived the longest.* Washington, D.C.: National Geographic.

Bunner, A. E., Agarwal, U., Gonzales, J. F., Valente, F.; Barnard, N. D. (2014). Nutrition intervention for migraine: A randomized crossover trial. *The Journal of Headache and Pain, 15*(1). doi:10.1186/1129-2377-15-69

Burke, E. (n.d.). Edmund Burke Quotes. Retrieved January 26, 2021, from https://www.brainyquote.com/quotes/edmund_burke_103841

Chai, N. C., Peterlin, B. L., & Calhoun, A. H. (2014). Migraine and estrogen. *Current Opinion in Neurology, 27*(3), 315–324. https://doi.org/10.1097/WCO.0000000000000091

Chao, A., Grilo, C. M., White, M. A., & Sinha, R. (2015). Food cravings mediate the relationship between chronic stress and body mass index. *Journal of Health Psychology, 20*(6), 721–729. https://doi.org/10.1177/1359105315573448

Chopra, D., M.D. (2013, June 12). Healing Wisdom. Retrieved September 06, 2020, from https://chopra.com/articles/healing-wisdom

Cloud, H. (2011). Necessary endings: The employees, businesses, and relationships that all of us have to give up in order to move forward. New York, NY: HarperCollins.

Cook, C. J., & Jones, D. (2008). Hemiplegic migraine associated with interscalene block and general anaesthesia. *Anaesthesia, 63*(6), 678-679. doi:10.1111/j.1365-2044.2008.05555.x

Couvineau, A., Ceraudo, E., Tan, Y. V., Nicole, P., & Laburthe, M. (2012). The VPAC1 receptor: structure and function of a class B GPCR prototype. *Frontiers in Endocrinology, 3*, 139. https://doi.org/10.3389/fendo.2012.00139

Dahri, M., Tarighat-Esfanjani, A., Asghari-Jafarabadi, M., & Hashemilar, M. (2018). Oral coenzyme Q10 supplementation in patients with migraine: effects on clinical features and inflammatory markers, *Nutritional Neuroscience*, doi: 10.1080/1028415X.2017.1421039

Davis, J. L., Paris, H. L., Beals, J. W., Binns, S. E., Giordano, G. R., Scalzo, R. L., Schweder, M. M., Blair, E., & Bell, C. (2016). Liposomal-encapsulated ascorbic acid: influence on vitamin c bioavailability and capacity to protect against ischemia-reperfusion injury. *Nutrition and Metabolic Insights, 9*, 25–30. https://doi.org/10.4137/NMI.S39764

Dias, B. G., & Ressler, K. J. (2014). Parental olfactory experience influences behavior and neural structure in subsequent generations. *Nature Neuroscience, 17*(1), 89–96. https://doi.org/10.1038/nn.3594

Dowdle, H. (2010, January 14). Find Balance with the Four Aims of Life. Retrieved September 21, 2020, from https://www.yogajournal.com/yoga-101/aim-high

Drummond, P. D. (2006). Tryptophan depletion increases nausea, headache and photophobia in migraine sufferers. *Cephalalgia: An International Journal of Headache, 26*(10), 1225–1233. https://doi.org/10.1111/j.1468-2982.2006.01212.x

Durham, P. L. (2006). Calcitonin Gene-Related Peptide (CGRP) and Migraine. Headache: *The Journal of Head and Face Pain, 46*(S1). doi:10.1111/j.1526-4610.2006.00483.x

Emmanuella-King, K., & Ashe, A. (2017, August 11). Start Where You Are. Use What You Have. Do What You Can. Retrieved October 19, 2020, from http://kobiemmanuella-king.com/start-where-you-are-use-what-you-have-do-what-you-can/

Evcili, G., Utku, U., Öğün, M. N., & Özdemir, G. (2018). Early and long period follow-up results of low glycemic index diet for migraine prophylaxis. *The Journal of the Turkish Society of Algology, 30*(1), 8–11. https://doi.org/10.5505/agri.2017.62443

Evening Primrose Oil. (2016). Retrieved June 22, 2020, from https://www.nccih.nih.gov/health/evening-primrose-oil

Faraguna, U., Nelson, A., Vyazovskiy, V. V., Cirelli, C., & Tononi, G. (2010). Unilateral cortical spreading depression affects sleep need and induces molecular and electrophysiological signs of synaptic potentiation in vivo. *Cerebral Cortex, 20*(12), 2939-2947. doi:10.1093/cercor/bhq041

Geraghty, A. A., Lindsay, K. L., Alberdi, G., McAuliffe, F. M., & Gibney, E. R. (2016). Nutrition During Pregnancy Impacts Offspring's Epigenetic Status-Evidence from Human and Animal Studies. *Nutrition and Metabolic Insights, 8*(Suppl 1), 41–47. https://doi.org/10.4137/NMI.S29527

Ghorbani, Z., Rafiee, P., Fotouhi, A., Haghighi, S., Rasekh Magham, R., Ahmadi, Z. S., Djalali, M., Zareei, M., Razeghi Jahromi, S., Shahemi, S., Mahmoudi, M., & Togha, M. (2020). The effects of vitamin D supplementation on interictal serum levels of calcitonin gene-related peptide (CGRP) in episodic migraine patients: post hoc analysis of a randomized double-blind placebo-controlled trial. *The Journal of Headache and Pain, 21*(1), 22. https://doi.org/10.1186/s10194-020-01090-w

Godek, D. (2019, February 21). Physiology, Diving Reflex. Retrieved June 15, 2020, from https://www.ncbi.nlm.nih.gov/books/NBK538245/

Gorvett, Z. (2018, August 6). How the menstrual cycle changes women's brains – for better. Retrieved August 15, 2020, from https://www.bbc.com/future/article/20180806-how-the-menstrual-cycle-changes-womens-brains-every-month

Goschorska, M., Gutowska, I., Baranowska-Bosiacka, I., Barczak, K., & Chlubek, D. (2020). The use of antioxidants in the treatment of migraine. *Antioxidants (Basel, Switzerland), 9*(2), 116. https://doi.org/10.3390/antiox9020116

Gosseries, O. (2018). Neuroimaging Studies on Yoga Practice in Healthy Population. *Journal Yoga & Physiotherapy, 6*(2): 555681. DOI: 10.19080/JYP.2018.06.555681.

Greco, R., Demartini, C., Zanaboni, A. M., Piomelli, D., & Tassorelli, C. (2018). Endocannabinoid System and Migraine Pain: An Update. *Frontiers in Neuroscience, 12*, 172. https://doi.org/10.3389/fnins.2018.00172

Hales, C., Carroll, M., Fryar, C., & Ogden, C. (2020, February 27). Products - Data Briefs - Number 360 - February 2020. Retrieved July 07, 2020, from https://www.cdc.gov/nchs/products/databriefs/db360.htm

Harriott, A.M., Takizawa, T., Chung, D.Y. et al. (2019). Spreading depression as a preclinical model of migraine. *Journal of Headache Pain 20, 45.* https://doi.org/10.1186/s10194-019-1001-4

Herman, J. P., McKlveen, J. M., Ghosal, S., Kopp, B., Wulsin, A., Makinson, R., Scheimann, J., & Myers, B. (2016). Regulation of the hypothalamic-pituitary-adrenocortical stress response. *Comprehensive Physiology, 6*(2), 603–621. https://doi.org/10.1002/cphy.c150015

Holland, P.R., Barloese, M. & Fahrenkrug, J. (2018). PACAP in hypothalamic regulation of sleep and circadian rhythm: importance for headache. *Journal of Headache Pain 19, 20.* https://doi.org/10.1186/s10194-018-0844-4

Huff T., Daly D.T. Neuroanatomy, cranial nerve 5 (Trigeminal) [Updated 2020 May 23]. In: StatPearls [Internet]. Treasure Island (FL): StatPearls Publishing; 2020 Jan. Available from: https://www.ncbi.nlm.nih.gov/books/NBK482283/

Hussein, M., Fathy, W., Abd Elkareem, RM. (2019). The potential role of serum vitamin D level in migraine headache: a case–control study. *Journal of Pain Research.* 12:2529-2536 https://doi.org/10.2147/JPR.S216314

Institute for Health Metrics and Evaluation (IHME). (2018). *Findings from the Global Burden of Disease Study 2017.* Retrieved June 2, 2020.

Iyengar, B. K. (2014). Yoga: The path to holistic health. London: DK.

Jacobs, B., & Dussor, G. (2016). Neurovascular contributions to migraine: Moving beyond vasodilation. *Neuroscience, 338,* 130–144. https://doi.org/10.1016/j.neuroscience.2016.06.012

Jensen, M. T., Suadicani, P., Hein, H. O., and Gyntelberg, F. (2013). Elevated resting heart rate, physical fitness and all-cause mortality: A 16-year follow-up in the Copenhagen Male Study. *Heart, 99*(12), 882-887. doi:10.1136/heartjnl-2012-303375

Kiecolt-Glaser, J. K., Christian, L., Preston, H., Houts, C. R., Malarkey, W. B., Emery, C. F., & Glaser, R. (2010). Stress, inflammation, and yoga practice. *Psychosomatic Medicine, 72*(2), 113–121. https://doi.org/10.1097/PSY.0b013e3181cb9377

Kok, B. E., & Fredrickson, B. L. (2010). Upward spirals of the heart: Autonomic flexibility, as indexed by vagal tone, reciprocally and prospectively predicts positive emotions and social connectedness. *Biological Psychology, 85*(3), 432-436. doi: 10.1016/j.biopsycho.2010.09.005

Lao Tzu Quotes. (n.d.). BrainyQuote.com. Retrieved March 14, 2021, from https://www.brainyquote.com/quotes/lao_tzu_121075

Leimuranta, P., Khiroug, L., & Giniatullin, R. (2018). Emerging role of (endo)cannabinoids in migraine. *Frontiers in Pharmacology, 9,* 420. https://doi.org/10.3389/fphar.2018.00420

Leonel, A. J., & Alvarez-Leite, J. I. (2012). Butyrate: implications for intestinal function. *Current Opinion in Clinical Nutrition and Metabolic Care, 15*(5), 474–479. https://doi.org/10.1097/MCO.0b013e32835665fa

Lipton, R.B., Göbel H., Einhäupl, K.M., Wilks, K., Mauskop, A. (2004). Petasites hybridus root (butterbur) is an effective preventive treatment for migraine. *Neurology, 63*(12):2240-4.

Marashly, E. T., & Bohlega, S. A. (2017). Riboflavin has neuroprotective potential: focus on Parkinson's disease and migraine. *Frontiers in Neurology, 8*, 333. https://doi.org/10.3389/fneur.2017.00333

Marci, D., & Aberman, D. (2019, April 12). Magnesium and Migraine. Retrieved September 04, 2020, from https://www.migrainestrong.com/magnesium-and-migraine/

Martins-Oliveira, M., Akerman, S., Tavares, I., & Goadsby, P. (2017). Neuropeptide Y inhibits the trigeminovascular pathway through NPY Y1 receptor. *Pain, 158*(4), 765. doi: 10.1097/j.pain.0000000000000900

Mauskop A., Altura B.T, Altura B.M. (2001). Serum ionized magnesium in serum ionized calcium/ionized magnesium ratios in women with menstrual migraine. *Headache.* 42, 242–248.

Mccall, M. C. (2013). How might yoga work? An overview of potential underlying mechanisms. *Journal of Yoga; Physical Therapy, 03*(01). doi:10.4172/2157-7595.1000130

McCorry L. K. (2007). Physiology of the autonomic nervous system. *American Journal of Pharmaceutical Education, 71*(4), 78. https://doi.org/10.5688/aj710478

Meng, J., Ovsepian, S. V., Wang, J., Pickering, M., Sasse, A., Aoki, K. R., Dolly, J. O. (2009). Activation of trpv1 mediates calcitonin gene-related peptide release, which excites trigeminal sensory neurons and is attenuated by a retargeted botulinum toxin with anti-nociceptive potential. *Journal of Neuroscience, 29*(15), 4981-4992. doi:10.1523/jneurosci.5490-08.2009

Migraine Management Approaches: Science of Migraine. (2020). Retrieved June 11, 2020, from https://www.scienceofmigraine.com/cgrp-and-its-receptors/

Mitochondria [Digital image]. (2019, April 12). Retrieved September 02, 2020, from Removal of Damaged Mitochondria Helps Treat Chronic Inflammatory Disease. (2019, April 12). https://www.genengnews.com/news/removal-of-damaged-mitochondria-helps-treat-chronic-inflammatory-disease/

Mody, J. (2018) Epigenetics and yoga. *Journal of Clinical Epigenetics, 4*(2)10.

Murphy J,. Heptinstall S., Mitchell J. (1988). Randomized, double-blind, placebo-controlled trial of feverfew in migraine prevention. *Lancet.* 2:189-192.

Naghibi, M. M., Day, R., Stone, S., & Harper, A. (2019). Probiotics for the prophylaxis of migraine: a systematic review of randomized placebo-controlled trials. *Journal of Clinical Medicine, 8*(9), 1441. https://doi.org/10.3390/jcm8091441

Namkung, H., Kim, S. H., & Sawa, A. (2017). The Insula: an underestimated brain area in clinical neuroscience, psychiatry, and neurology. *Trends in Neurosciences, 40*(4), 200–207. https://doi.org/10.1016/j.tins.2017.02.002

Nooten, B. A., & Holland, G. B. (1994). Rig Veda: A metrically restored text with an introduction and notes. Cambridge, MA: Publ. by the Department of Sanskrit and Indian Studies, Harvard University.

O'Donnell, K. (2020). *The everyday Ayurveda guide to self-care: Rhythms, routines, and home remedies for natural healing.* Boulder, CO: Shambhala.

Office of Dietary Supplements - Riboflavin. (2020, June 3). Retrieved June 28, 2020, from https://ods.od.nih.gov/factsheets/Riboflavin-HealthProfessional/

Parohan, M., Sarraf, P., Javanbakht, M. H., Ranji-Burachaloo, S., & Djalali, M. (2019). Effect of coenzyme Q10 supplementation on clinical features of migraine: A systematic review and dose–response meta-analysis of randomized controlled trials. *Nutritional Neuroscience,* 1-8. doi:10.1080/1028415x.2019.1572940

Plato, Jowett, B. (1892). *The dialogues of Plato.* Oxford: At the Clarendon Press.

Pradhan, G., Samson, S. L., & Sun, Y. (2013). Ghrelin: much more than a hunger hormone. *Current Opinion In Clinical Nutrition And Metabolic Care, 16*(6), 619–624. https://doi.org/10.1097/MCO.0b013e328365b9be

Price, S. (2020, January 20). CBD: Understanding how CBD works with our bodies. Retrieved June 22, 2020, from https://www.healtheuropa.eu/cbd-understanding-how-cbd-works-with-our-bodies/96718/

Quinn, A. (2020). Aidan Quinn. Retrieved August 31, 2020, from https://www.brainyquote.com/authors/aidan-quinn-quotes

Rabelais, F., & Fragonard, M. (2009). *Pantagruel.* Paris: Pocket.

Removal of Damaged Mitochondria Helps Treat Chronic Inflammatory Disease. (2019, April 12). Retrieved September 02, 2020, from https://www.genengnews.com/news/removal-of-damaged-mitochondria-helps-treat-chronic-inflammatory-disease/

Rowe, J., & Kahn, R. (1987). Human aging: Usual and successful. *Science, 237*(4811), 143-149. doi:10.1126/science.3299702

Salehi, B., Sharopov, F., Fokou, P., Kobylinska, A., Jonge, L., Tadio, K., Sharifi-Rad, J., Posmyk, M. M., Martorell, M., Martins, N., & Iriti, M. (2019). Melatonin in medicinal and food plants: occurrence, bioavailability, and health potential for humans. *Cells, 8*(7), 681. https://doi.org/10.3390/cells8070681

Sastri, A. M., & Sankaracharya. (2004). The Bhagavad Gita. Madras: Samata Books.

Schieber, M., & Chandel, N. S. (2014). ROS function in redox signaling and oxidative stress. *Current Biology, 24*(10), R453–R462. https://doi.org/10.1016/j.cub.2014.03.034

Schoenen J., Jacquy J., Lenaerts M. (1998). Effectiveness of high-dose riboflavin in migraine prophylaxis: a randomized controlled trial. *Neurology.* 50:466-470.

Seligman, M. (2018). Mihaly Csikszentmihalyi. Retrieved September 09, 2020, from https://www.pursuit-of-happiness.org/history-of-happiness/mihaly-csikszentmihalyi/

Shakespeare, W., Barnes, S., & Coleman, A. (2017). *William Shakespeare's Macbeth*. Cheltenham, Victoria: Insight Publications.

Skaper, S. D., & Di Marzo, V. (2012). Endocannabinoids in nervous system health and disease: the big picture in a nutshell. *Philosophical Transactions of the Royal Society of London. Series B, Biological Sciences, 367*(1607), 3193–3200. https://doi.org/10.1098/rstb.2012.0313

Sohl, S. J., Birdee, G., & Elam, R. (2016). Complementary tools to empower and sustain behavior change: motivational interviewing and mindfulness. *American Journal of Lifestyle Medicine, 10*(6), 429–436. https://doi.org/10.1177/1559827615571524

Sprenger, T., Viana, M., & Tassorelli, C. (2018). Current prophylactic medications for migraine and their potential mechanisms of action, neurotherapeutics. *The Journal of the American Society for Experimental NeuroTherapeutics, 15*(2), 313–323. https://doi.org/10.1007/s13311-018-0621-8

Sterling K. Brown Quotes. (n.d.). BrainyQuote.com. Retrieved March 14, 2021, from https://www.brainyquote.com/quotes/sterling_k_brown_775174

Strother, L. C., Srikiatkhachorn, A., & Supronsinchai, W. (2018). Targeted orexin and hypothalamic neuropeptides for migraine. Neurotherapeutics. *Journal of the American Society for Experimental NeuroTherapeutics, 15*(2), 377–390. https://doi.org/10.1007/s13311-017-0602-3

Tepper, D., MD. (2013). Magnesium and migraine prevention. Retrieved July 09, 2020, from https://americanmigrainefoundation.org/resource-library/magnesium/

Timoszuk, M., Bielawska, K., & Skrzydlewska, E. (2018). Evening primrose (oenothera biennis) biological activity dependent on chemical composition. *Antioxidants* (Basel, Switzerland), *7*(8), 108. https://doi.org/10.3390/antiox7080108

Trivieri, L. (2006). The American Holistic Medical Association guide to holistic health: Healing therapies for optimal wellness. New York, NY: Wiley.

Vallath N. (2010). Perspectives on yoga inputs in the management of chronic pain. *Indian Journal of Palliative Care, 16*(1), 1–7. https://doi.org/10.4103/0973-1075.63127

Values list. (2020). Retrieved September 11, 2020, from https://eleducation.org/

Villemure, C., Ceko, M., Cotton, V. A., & Bushnell, M. C. (2014). Insular cortex mediates increased pain tolerance in yoga practitioners. *Cerebral Cortex, 24*(10), 2732–2740. https://doi.org/10.1093/cercor/bht124

What is Newton's first law? (article). (2020). Retrieved August 02, 2020, from https://www.khanacademy.org/science/physics/forces-newtons-laws/newtons-laws-of-motion/a/what-is-newtons-first-law

Wolf, J. (2016, November 27). Heal your headache with Ayurveda. Retrieved October 12, 2020, from https://www.thelotusroomnashville.com/living-ayurveda/2016/11/27/heal-your-headache-with-ayurveda

Ziaei, S., Kazemnejad, A., & Sedighi, A. (2009). The effect of vitamin E on the treatment of menstrual migraine. *Medical Science Monitor: International Medical Journal of Experimental And Clinical Research, 15*(1), CR16–CR19.

Zopa, L. Z. (2018). Four Noble Truths: A Guide to Everyday Life. Wisdom Publications.

Author Biography

A refreshing deviation to the standard, Elizabeth Priller lives out her vision for transforming the way people live and work. She is the founder of Elizabeth Priller Consulting and Locus Coworking Wellness Space based out of Northwest Illinois. In her contributions as a Corporate Wellness, Diversity, Equity, and Inclusion Consultant, she partners with leaders and educators worldwide to optimize how their teams think, breathe, move, eat, and sleep. Elizabeth facilitates how to move out of chronically stressed bodies and minds in order to thrive in life and work.

Spending the first ten years of her life in Southside Chicago, Elizabeth was abruptly uprooted and replanted in a rural Midwest town of 600 people in the early 90s. Coupled with this drastic cultural shift, she took an uncommon path to her career - starting nursing school as a teen mother. For over 24 years, Elizabeth lived and worked in what she thought was normal: burned out, not sleeping well, in a constant state of inflammation, and without a distinct purpose. She eventually flipped the script of a quasi-common practice: that work has to be a mindless run on the hamster wheel. She now helps people see that work can be an unrepeatable expression of individual purpose, that is fulfilled through a well mind and body.

In the last two decades of experience as a Registered Nurse, Certified Health Coach, Registered Yoga Teacher, Certified Ayurvedic Specialist, and educator, she has earned several excellence and leadership awards at the local, regional, and national level. In 2017, she was awarded the ACTE Illinois and Region III New Teacher of the Year and was nominated as a national finalist.

Her ethos, "The body follows the mind" is the basis of her recently published book, *The Migraine Method: The Steps to a Migraine-Free Life Through Science and Spirituality.* Elizabeth helps shine a light on how value-based transformation contributes to improved well-being and a clear sense of purpose. She believes that a thriving life is at the intersection of resilience-empowered transformation.

To fill her own cup, Elizabeth thrives on solo travel, flying airplanes, practicing yoga, spending time in her garden with bees and butterflies, and creating memories with her husband, daughters, and grandson.

You can find the results of how she transforms the way people live and work at **www.elizabethpriller.com.**

Notes

Made in the USA
Monee, IL
11 January 2022

87414629R10236